Get Through

Accident and Emergency Medicine:
MCQs

D0994549

Get Through
Accident and Emergency
Medicine: MCQs

Amy Herlihy MBChB MRCS(Edin) BaO BSc

The ROYAL
SOCIETY *of*
MEDICINE
PRESS *Limited*

© 2007 Royal Society of Medicine Press Ltd

Published by the Royal Society of Medicine Press Ltd
1 Wimpole Street, London W1G 0AE, UK
Tel: +44 (0)20 7290 2921
Fax: +44 (0)20 7290 2929
E-mail: publishing@rsm.ac.uk
Website: www.rsmpress.co.uk

British Library Cataloguing in Publication Data
A catalogue record for this book is available from the British Library

ISBN 1-85315-694-9

Distribution in Europe and Rest of World:

Marston Book Services Ltd

PO Box 269
Abingdon
Oxon OX14 4YN, UK
Tel: +44 (0)1235 465500
Fax: +44 (0)1235 465555
Email: direct.order@marston.co.uk

Distribution in the USA and Canada:

Royal Society of Medicine Press Ltd
c/o BookMasters, Inc.
30 Amberwood Parkway
Ashland, Ohio 44805, USA
Tel: +1 800 247 6553/ +1 800 266 5564
Fax: +1 419 281 6883
Email: order@bookmasters.com

Distribution in Australia and New Zealand:

Elsevier Australia
30-52 Smidmore Street
Marrikville NSW 2204, Australia
Tel: +61 2 9349 5811
Fax: +61 2 9349 5911
Email: service@elsevier.com.au

Typeset by Phoenix Photosetting, Chatham, Kent, UK
Printed and bound by Bell & Bain Ltd, Glasgow, UK

Contents

Abbreviations

ABG	arterial blood gas
ACE	angiotensin-converting enzyme
ACTH	adrenocorticotrophic hormone
AIDS	acquired immune deficiency syndrome
ALT	alanine aminotransferase
AST	aspartate transaminase
BP	blood pressure
CMV	cytomegalovirus
COPD	chronic obstructive pulmonary disease
CSF	cerebrospinal fluid
CT	computed tomography
CTPA	CT pulmonary angiogram
CVA	cerebrovascular accident
CVP	central venous pressure
CXR	chest X-ray
DIC	disseminated intravascular coagulation
DPL	diagnostic peritoneal lavage
ECG	electrocardiogram
ET	endotracheal
FEV_1	forced expiratory volume in 1 second
GGT	gamma-glytamyl transpeptidase
GTN	glycerol trinitrate
HATI	human antitetanus immunoglobulin
HELLP	haemolysis, elevated liver enzymes, low platelets
HIV	human immunodeficiency virus
ICP	intracranial pressure
IPPV	intermittent positive pressure ventilation
ITU	intensive treatment unit
IV	intravenous
IVU	intravenous urethrogram
JVP	jugular venous pressure
LDH	lactate dehydrogenase
MC&S	microscopy, culture and sensitivity
MEN	multiple endocrine neoplasia
NAI	nonaccidental injury
NSAID	nonsteroidal anti-inflammatory drug
PCP	*Pneumocystis carinii* pneumonia
PEF	peak expiratory flow
POP	plaster of Paris
PSVT	premature supraventricular tachycardia
Rbc	red blood cells
SBP	systolic blood pressure
SIADH	syndrome of inappropriate ADH secretion
STD	sexually transmitted disease

TB	tuberculosis
TCA	tricyclic antidepressant
Wbc	white blood cells
Wcc	white cell count
WPW	Wolff–Parkinson–White syndrome

Introduction

As anyone who has ever sat an MCQ style examination knows, practising MCQs is invaluable preparation for exam success. It not only provides you with new information but also teaches you techniques in how to answer the questions. You learn the tricks of double negative questions, the importance of reading every word with care, and the type of details needed to pass that you may otherwise skim over.

Unfortunately when I sat the MRCS A&E examination there were no practice MCQ books available that dealt with my chosen specialty. I found it frustrating studying for an MCQ style examination without the help of any practice books. Hopefully this book will stop all those studying for the examination in the future from feeling the same way. If you have already passed the examination it will provide you with a useful revision aid when brushing up on topics that you may not have read about for a while.

There are currently two colleges that hold A&E examinations. The Royal College of Surgeons Edinburgh hosts this examination biannually and the College of Emergency Medicine hosts a similar style exam. This MCQ book is designed to help you prepare for both of these examinations. Successful completion of either examination allows you to progress to Higher Specialist Training in Accident and Emergency Medicine.

Book format

The book groups questions by subject to allow for easy revision before the examination. These cover the wide range of specialties seen as an A&E clinician, including orthopaedics, trauma, acute medicine, paediatrics, surgery, toxicology, ophthalmology, gynaecology, infectious disease, and anatomy. With over 400 questions there is large scope to study and refine your knowledge before the examination.

The anatomy section is based on the syllabus as outlined by the College of Emergency Medicine. All questions are based on current guidelines regarding the practise of A&E medicine.

Explanations are provided with the answers to aid understanding of the subject matter.

Examination format

Royal College of Surgeons Edinburgh

The examination comprises an MCQ paper, an oral examination, and a clinical component. To be eligible to sit this examination you must hold Part 1 of either the MCRP or MRCPCH, the MCQ component of the MRCS or part A of the Membership of the College of Emergency Medicine.

The MCQ paper lasts for 2 hours and contains 60 questions, each with five stems (and this is the style used here, with the exception of the ABG MCQs). It tests the candidate's knowledge in the applied basic sciences and the principles of A&E medicine and surgery in general. There is negative marking: questions are scored on the basis of +1 for a correct answer and –1 for a wrong answer.

The oral examination consists of two 20-minute orals. One is based on surgery in A&E medicine, the other on medicine in A&E medicine.

The candidate progresses to the clinical component upon successful completion of both the MCQ and oral sections.

College of Emergency Medicine

Part A consists of 50 MCQs, each with four stems. It is not negatively marked. It examines basic sciences as applied to emergency medicine. Candidates must pass Part A before proceeding to Part B.

Part B examines data interpretation skills.

Part C consists of 18 Objective Structured Clinical Examination (OSCE) stations.

Examination techniques

1. Read the whole paper before answering anything. This allows you to start subconsciously recalling subject matter in advance of answering the questions.
2. Read every word carefully. MCQs are often answered incorrectly because a double negative is misread or the stems are not read fully before the question is answered. Some stems contain both correct and incorrect information which can easily catch a candidate out if the question is not read thouroughly.
3. For the MRCS A&E examination count how many questions you have answered. Remember that there is negative marking so you will need to consider how many questions you need to answer to pass.
4. For the College of Emergency Medicine examination there is no negative marking. Therefore answer all questions. Marks can be gained by guessing in this examination!
5. Mark the answer sheet carefully. Rubbers are provided by examination centres so ensure that all wrong answers are carefully erased. These papers are machine read and answers need to be clearly marked to be interpreted correctly.
6. Time yourself. Ensure you are allowing enough time to get through each question in the paper. Generally each question contains at least one easy stem and these provide a valuable opportunity for picking up marks.
7. Read terms such as 'commonly' 'usually' or 'all' carefully as they may change a question's meaning. A rare disease may cause a specific sign but may not be a common cause of it! Questions including the term 'all' are more often negative than positive. As all doctors know there are very few absolutes in medicine.

Finally, good luck with the examination!

I. Trauma

1.1 The following are IV induction agents:

    a. Thiopentone
    b. Propofol
    c. Vecuronium
    d. Atracurium
    e. Ketamine

1.2 Regarding muscle relaxants:

    a. Suxamethonium is a short-acting non-depolarizing muscle relaxant
    b. Suxamethonium causes raised intraocular pressure
    c. Suxamethonium may cause hyperkalaemia
    d. Suxamethonium is contraindicated in crush injuries
    e. Suxamethonium acts for approximately 20–30 minutes

1.3 Increased risk of lignocaine toxicity is associated with:

    a. Heart block
    b. Elderly patients
    c. Phaeochromocytoma
    d. Beta-blockers
    e. Cimetidine

1.4 Regarding local anaesthetic nerve blocks:

    a. Digital nerve block requires a single injection
    b. In median nerve block the needle should be inserted between the palmaris longus and flexor carpi radialis
    c. Carpal tunnel syndrome is not a contraindication to median nerve blockade at the wrist joint
    d. Infraorbital nerve block is used to anaesthetize the lower lip
    e. Supraorbital nerve block is safe to administer

1.5 Regarding lignocaine and adrenaline:

    a. Should be avoided in patients with ischaemic heart disease
    b. Safe to use in patients with phaeochromocytoma
    c. Safe to use in diabetic patients
    d. Contraindicated for use in children
    e. Should be used with caution in patients on beta-blockers

1.6 Regarding Bier's blockade:

a. Recommended for surgery lasting less than 45 minutes
b. Useful in patients with peripheral vascular disease
c. Bupivacaine is the anaesthetic drug of choice
d. An IV cannula should be inserted bilaterally
e. Tourniquet should be inflated to 50 mmHg above the systolic blood pressure

1.7 Regarding suxamethonium:

a. Contraindicated in open globe injury
b. Contraindicated in hepatic failure
c. Hyperkalaemia is a recognized side-effect
d. Rhabdomyolysis is a recognized side-effect
e. It is an anaesthetic induction agent

1.8 Entonox contraindications:

a. Temperatures below −6 °C
b. Base of skull fracture
c. Pneumothorax
d. Temperatures above 30 °C
e. After diving

1.9 Regarding ketamine:

a. Causes hypertension
b. Causes tachycardia
c. Can cause hallucinations
d. Acts as a bronchoconstrictor
e. Contraindicated in people with phaeochromocytoma

1.10 Nasal diamorphine contraindications:

a. Weight < 15 kg
b. Base skull fracture
c. Age under 5 years
d. Nasal polyps
e. Nasal bone fracture

1.11 Head injury:

a. All patients on warfarin should be referred to hospital
b. Children rarely have serious head injury without a skull fracture
c. Skull X-ray should be performed on patients with a Glasgow Coma Scale of 12
d. Irritable patients with a Glasgow Coma Scale of 15 can be safely discharged
e. Patients with amnesia post head injury should be managed by their GP

1.12 **Regarding head trauma and uncal herniation:**

    a. Intracranial pressure of 30 mmHg is normal
    b. Cerebral blood flow of 50 ml/100 g brain/min is normal
    c. Complete cranial nerve III paralysis causes the eye to face down and inwards
    d. Ipsilateral limb weakness occurs
    e. Pupillary dilation occurs on the same side as the lesion

1.13 **Regarding pupillary sizes:**

    a. Pontine lesions cause bilateral dilated pupils
    b. Opioids cause bilateral constricted pupils
    c. Optic nerve damage causes a unilateral constricted pupil
    d. Carotid sheath damage causes a unilateral dilated pupil
    e. Inadequate brain perfusion causes bilateral dilated pupils

1.14 **Subdural haematoma:**

    a. Has a concave appearance on CT scanning
    b. Usually associated with a clear history of head injury
    c. Increased risk with age
    d. Extensor response to pain indicates a good prognosis
    e. Usually easy to distinguish clinically from an extradural haematoma

1.15 **Regarding imaging in head injuries:**

    a. Patients with neurological dysfunction should have a skull X-ray
    b. A fluid level in the sphenoid sinus indicates a skull fracture
    c. 1-mm shift of the pineal gland indicates probable intracranial haemorrhage
    d. Loss of integrity of the craniocervical junction indicates a skull fracture
    e. All patients with plain film evidence of skull fracture require a CT brain

1.16 **Regarding extradural haematoma:**

    a. Middle ear infection may cause this
    b. A dural sinus tear is the most common cause
    c. Skull fractures are present in < 80% of adult cases
    d. Often have no lucid interval before coma
    e. May cause an extensor plantar response

1.17 **Regarding the treatment of raised intracranial pressure:**

    a. Mannitol is used in management
    b. Corticosteroids are not used if the rise in pressure is secondary to a space- occupying lesion
    c. Pyrexia may cause cerebral vasodilatation
    d. Treatment involves lowering the head of the bed
    e. Treatment involves cooling the patient to 35 °C

1.18 Regarding facial trauma:

a. Major cause of death is asphyxia
b. Bleeding is usually from branches of the internal carotid artery
c. The zygoma is the most common facial bone to fracture
d. Isolated maxillary fractures are rare
e. The mandible has a high incidence of multiple fractures

1.19 Regarding Glasgow Coma Scale:

a. Glasgow Coma Scale 12 = eyes opening, speech verbally confused and localizing pain
b. Glasgow Coma Scale 7 = eyes opening, speech, incomprehensible sounds, and abnormal flexion to pain
c. Is an international scale from 0 to 15 indicating neurological status
d. Coma is defined as a Glasgow Coma Scale of < 9
e. Should be used with caution if patient younger than 5 years old

1.20 Ocular injury:

a. Hyphaema is treated by surgical drainage
b. Hyphaema is associated with secondary glaucoma
c. A hyphaema covering greater than two-thirds of the iris can damage the drainage angle
d. Ciliary prolapse indicates penetration injury
e. Corneal injury from a penetrating injury has a poor prognosis

1.21 Facial nerve palsy:

a. Upper motor neuron injuries spare the forehead
b. Bell's palsy involves cranial nerves VI, VII, and VIII
c. Otitis media can cause a facial nerve palsy
d. Herpes zoster may cause a Bell's palsy
e. Injury at the stylomastoid foramen causes loss of taste and hyperacusis

1.22 Regarding opthalmolgical trauma:

a. Hyphaema is associated with penetrating trauma
b. Proptosis occurs with orbital floor fracture
c. Nose blowing is a useful diagnostic aid in facial fracture
d. Alkalis cause more serious eye injuries than acids
e. Corneoscleral wounds are most commonly located superiorly

1.23 Regarding Le Fort facial fracture:

a. Describes fractures through the mid portion of the face
b. Associated with altered pupil levels
c. Is a recognized cause of diplopia
d. Le Fort 3 describes fracture through the sinus wall laterally and nasal bones medially
e. Le Fort 1 describes fractures detaching the palate and maxillary alveolus

1.24 Regarding initial trauma surveys:

a. Assessment for the presence of an open pneumothorax forms part of the primary survey

b. Assessment for the presence of a minor haemothorax forms part of the primary survey

c. Assessment for the presence of a tracheobronchial tree injury forms part of the secondary survey

d. Open pneumothorax should initially be treated with a fully occlusive dressing

e. Assessment for a traumatic simple pneumothorax is part of the secondary survey

1.25 Regarding spinal injuries:

a. Approximately 25% of patients with a vertebral fracture have a second vertebral fracture

b. It is associated with bradycardia and hypertension

c. Presence of priapism suggests quadriplegia

d. If methylprednisolone is used in management, treatment should be commenced 8 hours after injury

e. Chance fractures of the lumbar spine do not involve the intervertebral disc

1.26 Regarding cervical spine trauma:

a. Atlas fractures are associated with occipital pain

b. Cord injury at C6 causes paraplegia

c. Diaphragmatic injury is seen in lesions affecting C5 and above

d. Flexion/extension films are indicated if subluxation is seen on lateral C-spine X-ray

e. Unstable flexion and rotation injuries require traction and posterior fusion

1.27 Signs of spinal cord injury in patients with reduced Glasgow Coma Scale:

a. Priapism

b. Hypotension and tachycardia

c. Response to pain above the clavicle, not below

d. Diaphragmatic breathing

e. Extension not flexion at the elbow joint

1.28 Cardiac tamponade:

a. Is associated with aortic dissection

b. ECG leads are of low voltage

c. Chest X-ray always shows globular cardiomegaly

d. If suspected, needle pericardiocentesis should be performed immediately

e. Is associated with raised JVP, raised BP, and reduced heart sounds

1.29 Regarding aortic dissection:

a. Acute myocardial infarction is a recognized complication
b. Aortic valve incompetence is a recognized complication
c. Aortic dilatation of > 5 cm is an indication for surgical repair
d. Surgical repair is recommended for Type A (using Stanford and DeBakey classification)
e. Surgical intervention is indicated for Type B if there is ischaemic compromise of the renal system

1.30 Regarding aortic dissection:

a. It is associated with cocaine use
b. It causes distortion of the left main stem bronchus on CXR
c. Medical management includes use of beta-blockers
d. Medical management includes use of sodium nitroprusside
e. Hypertension predisposes to aortic dissection

1.31 Signs of aortic rupture on CXR:

a. Undisplaced nasogastric tube
b. Pleural capping
c. Fracture of lower three ribs
d. Loss of space between the aorta and pulmonary artery
e. Upward and leftward shift of the right main stem bronchus

1.32 Aortic dissection associations:

a. Hypertension
b. Bicuspid aortic valve
c. Ehlers–Danlos syndrome
d. Pregnancy
e. Pneumothorax

1.33 Pneumothorax associations:

a. Sarcoidosis
b. Cystic fibrosis
c. Crohn's disease
d. Addison's disease
e. Pneumocystis pneumonia

1.34 Regarding tension pneumothorax:

a. It is associated with decreased venous return
b. IV cannula for decompression should be inserted immediately below the second rib
c. Should be examined for during the primary survey
d. Causes increased inflation pressure in patients receiving IPPV
e. Causes tracheal deviation towards the affected side

1.35 Regarding tension pneumothorax:

a. Causes collapsed neck veins
b. Causes hyper-resonance of the affected side
c. Causes a tachycardia
d. Causes absent breath sounds on the unaffected side
e. Requires a CXR for definite diagnosis

1.36 Regarding cricothyroidotomy:

a. Can provide up to 45 minutes of oxygenation
b. Surgical cricothyroidotomy is contraindicated in those younger than 12 years old
c. There is a risk of vocal cord damage
d. Indicated if suspected mid facial fracture and airway compromise
e. Damage to the cricothyroid artery may occur

1.37 Regarding airway obstruction:

a. Jaw thrust manœuvre is used in patients with cervical spine injuries
b. End tidal CO_2 monitoring definitively confirms correct placement of the endotracheal tube
c. Tracheal intubation is indicated if there is suspected midfacial fracture and airway compromise
d. Lateral neck X-rays should be preformed in cases of acute airway obstruction
e. Patients with increased intracranial pressure require intubation

1.38 Pulse oximetry is unreliable in:

a. Severe anaemia
b. An ill-fitting blood pressure cuff on the opposite limb
c. Carboxyhaemoglobinaemia
d. Methaemoglobinaemia
e. Thalassaemia

1.39 Nasotracheal intubation contraindications:

a. Age younger than 12 years old
b. Apnoea
c. Le Fort 2 facial fracture
d. Epistaxis
e. Nasal piercing

1.40 Regarding acute upper airway obstruction:

a. In epiglottitis severe respiratory distress is evident
b. Croup is associated with a very painful throat
c. Hypoxia is a useful early indicator of impending obstruction
d. Nebulized adrenaline is useful in children with mild croup
e. A 5-day course of prednisolone is given to children with croup

1.41 Regarding trauma while pregnant:

a. Associated with an increased risk of severe retroperitoneal haemorrhage
b. Associated with a decreased risk of pituitary infarction
c. Chest drains should be inserted one to two intercostal spaces higher than usual
d. Hypoxia develops slower than usual
e. Hypovolaemic shock shows delayed signs and symptoms

1.42 Regarding bullet and blast injuries:

a. Yaw describes the orientation of the longitudinal axis of the missile to its trajectory
b. In blast injuries the negative pressure phase lasts longer than the positive pressure phase
c. Secondary blast injury is when the person becomes the missile
d. Tertiary blast injury is due to flying objects
e. High velocity injuries usually require delayed primary closure

1.43 Indications for celiotomy:

a. Peritonitis post trauma
b. Haematemesis post penetrating trauma
c. > 250 Wbc/mm^3 on DPL
d. Hypotension post blunt trauma despite adequate resuscitation
e. > 100 000 Rbc/mm^3 on DPL

1.44 The following are characteristics of tetanus-prone wounds:

a. Wounds > 6 hours old
b. Crush injury
c. Burn injuries
d. Linear wounds
e. Depth of 0.5 cm

1.45 When treating patients with wounds:

a. All patients who have not had a tetanus vaccination should be given HATI
b. Pregnancy is a contraindication to tetanus vaccination
c. A history of a severe reaction to tetanus vaccination is a contraindication to administering HATI
d. A patient who has had six previous tetanus vaccinations should have another vaccination
e. Incubation period for tetanus is usually 4–14 days

1.46 Regarding hydrofluoric acid:

a. It is the inorganic acid of fluoride
b. Burns are associated with hypocalcaemia and hypomagnaesia
c. 20% solution causes immediate tissue destruction
d. Bier's blockade is useful for limb burns
e. Burns are associated with hypokalaemia

1.47 **Regarding hydrofluoric acid:**

   a. Burns can cause a systemic coagulopathy
   b. Intra-arterial $MgSO_4$ or intra-arterial calcium gluconate is
   used in management of severe burns
   c. Burns cause pain in proportion to the physical signs
   d. Irrigation is usually adequate treatment
   e. < 20% solution usually causes no tissue damage

1.48 **Regarding renal trauma:**

   a. A patient on glicazide may have an IVU
   b. A patient on metformin may have an IVU
   c. Absence of haematuria indicates no renal damage
   d. An IVU is indicated for frank haematuria
   e. A patient with myeloma may have an IVU

1.49 **Regarding needlestick injuries:**

   a. Risk of HIV transmission is approximately 10%
   b. Hepatitis C has higher rates of transmission than hepatitis B
   c. Post-exposure prophylaxis should be offered to all patients
   attending the A&E department
   d. Measures to prevent secondary transmission such as safe sex
   are not necessary after needlestick injury
   e. Negative hepatitis C titres at 6 months indicate disease-free
   status

1.1 Answers

a. **True**
b. **True**
c. **False** – vecuronium is a muscle relaxant
d. **False** – atracurium is a muscle relaxant
e. **True**

1.2 Answers

a. **False** – suxamethonium is a short-acting depolarizing muscle relaxant
b. **True**
c. **True**
d. **True** – due to the risk of hyperkalaemia
e. **False** – suxamethonium acts for approximately 5 minutes

1.3 Answers

a. **True**
b. **True**
c. **False**
d. **True** – due to increased risk of myocardial depression
e. **True** – cimetidine inhibits the metabolism of lignocaine

1.4 Answers

a. **False** – digital nerve block requires injections on both sides of the finger
b. **True**
c. **False** – carpal tunnel syndrome is a contraindication to median nerve block at the wrist joint
d. **False** –the infraorbital nerve supplies sensation to the upper lip
e. **False** – supraorbital nerve block is not advisable as inadvertent injection into the orbit may cause temporary blindness if the anaesthetic reaches the optic nerve

1.5 Answers

a. **True**
b. **False** – lignocaine and adrenaline should not be used in patients with phaeochromocytoma
c. **True**
d. **False** – lignocaine and adrenaline may be used in children
e. **True** – beta-blockers predispose to increased risk of myocardial depression

1.6 Answers

a. **False** – Bier's blockade is used in procedures lasting < 30 minutes
b. **False** – peripheral vascular disease is a contraindication to use of Bier's blockade
c. **False** – prilocaine is used; bupivacaine is more likely to produce toxic reactions
d. **True** – an IV cannula is required in the opposite limb in case of emergency
e. **False** – tourniquet should be inflated to either 100 mmHg above the SBP or 300 mmHg

1.7 Answers

a. **True**
b. **False** – suxamethonium is contraindicated in acute renal failure
c. **True**
d. **True**
e. **False** – suxamethonium is a muscle relaxant

1.8 Answers

a. **True**
b. **True**
c. **True**
d. **False**
e. **True** – diving increases the risk of decompression illness

1.9 Answers

a. **True**
b. **True**
c. **True**
d. **False** – ketamine acts as a bronchodilator
e. **True** – due to risk of hypertension

1.10 Answers

a. **False** – weight < 10 kg is a contraindication to nasal diamorphine
b. **True**
c. **False** – nasal diamorphine is contraindicated in children younger than 1 year old
d. **True** – due to obstruction by the polyps
e. **True**

1.11 Answers

a. **True** – due to the risk of intracerebral haemorrhage
b. **False** – children commonly have serious head injury without a skull fracture, and hence skull X-rays are often unhelpful in the paediatric population
c. **False** – a Glasgow Coma Scale of 12 is an indication for CT brain
d. **False** – irritability warrants further investigation
e. **False** – all patients with amnesia post head injury should be referred to hospital

1.12 Answers

a. **False** – intracranial pressure of 10 mmHg is considered normal
b. **True**
c. **False** – complete cranial nerve III paralysis causes the eye to face downwards and outwards
d. **False** – contralateral limb weakness occurs due to involvement of the corticospinal tracts
e. **True** – due to parasympathetic pupillary constriction

1.13 Answers

a. **False** – pontine lesions cause bilateral constricted pupils
b. **True**
c. **False** – optic nerve damage causes dilated pupils bilaterally
d. **False** – carotid sheath damage causes injury to the sympathetic pathway and pupil constriction
e. **True**

1.14 Answers

a. **True**
b. **False** – if it is a chronic subdural haematoma the head injury is often so trivial it is not recalled
c. **True** – as cortical atrophy stretches bridging veins
d. **False** – extensor response to pain is a sign of a large haematoma and poor prognosis
e. **False** – usually very difficult to distinguish subdural and extradural haematomas clinically

1.15 Answers

a. **False** – neurological dysfunction is an indication for CT brain
b. **True**
c. **False** – a 3-mm shift of the pineal gland indicates probable intracranial haemorrhage
d. **True**
e. **True** – to rule out intracranial haemorrhage. The risk of haemorrhage increases from 1:100 to 1:30 in alert patients with skull fracture

1.16 Answers

a. **True**
b. **False** – dural sinus tear is a rare cause. A head injury causing tearing of the meningeal artery is the most common cause
c. **False** – skull fractures are present in > 90% of cases
d. **True**
e. **True**

1.17 Answers

a. **True**

b. **False** – corticosteroids are very useful in this instance as they may decrease the oedema surrounding the space-occupying lesion. Not used if the raised ICP is secondary to a cerebrovascular accident

c. **True** – thus increases cerebral metabolism

d. **False** – the head of the bed should be elevated to approx 30° degrees to promote venous drainage

e. **True** – to prevent cerebral ischaemia

1.18 Answers

a. **True** – due to upper airway obstruction

b. **False** – the external carotid artery branches cause bleeding except for at the nose, which has some supply from branches of the internal carotid artery

c. **False** – the nose is the most common site of fracture followed by the zygoma

d. **True**

e. **True** – due to its shape. The most common site of fracture is at the condylar neck and at the first or second molar

1.19 Answers

a. **True**

b. **True**

c. **False** – the scale is from 3 to 15

d. **True**

e. **True**

1.20 Answers

a. **False** – treatment for hyphaema is bed rest

b. **True** – if it is a total hyphaema

c. **True** – damage occurs at levels greater than one-third

d. **True**

e. **False** – corneal injury from a penetrating injury has a good prognosis; however, lens reimplantation may be required

1.21 Answers

a. **True**

b. **False** – Bell's palsy involves cranial nerve VII palsy in isolation. Acoustic neuroma may involve all three nerves

c. **True**

d. **False** – herpes zoster may cause a facial nerve palsy but not a Bell's palsy

e. **False** – injury at the petrous part of the temporal bone may cause loss of taste and hyperacusis

1.22 Answers

a. **True** – hyphaema may also occur after blunt eye injury
b. **True** – orbital floor fracture may cause a retrobulbar haemorrhage which in turn may cause proptosis to occur
c. **False** – nose blowing is dangerous as it can cause spread of infection intracranially
d. **True**
e. **False** – corneoscleral wounds are more often inferiorly located due to the upturning of the eye as the person blinks

1.23 Answers

a. **True**
b. **True**
c. **True**
d. **False** – this describes a Le Fort 2 fracture. A Le Fort 3 fracture involves the maxilla, zygoma, nasal bones, ethmoid, and the small bones of the base of the skull. The midface fractures from the base of the skull
e. **True**

1.24 Answers

a. **True**
b. **False** – assessment for the presence of a minor haemothorax is part of the secondary survey
c. **True**
d. **False** – a three-sided dressing is used to avoid causing a tension pneumothorax
e. **True**

1.25 Answers

a. **False** – approximately 10% of patients have a second vertebral fracture
b. **False** – peripheral vasodilatation causes hypotension. Due to interruption of the sympathetic nerve the vagus and parasympathetic nerves function unchecked causing a bradycardia
c. **True** – or a high midthoracic paraplegia
d. **False** – methylprednisolone should optimally be commenced within 8 hours of injury
e. **False** – Chance fracture causes horizontal splitting of the spinous process and neural arch, and extends into the superior posterior aspect of the vertebral body, and into and damaging the intervertebral disc

1.26 Answers

a. **True** – due to pressure on the great occipital nerve
b. **False** – cord injury at C6 causes quadriplegia
c. **True** – the diaphragm receives C3–C5 innervation
d. **False** – subluxation is a contraindication to lateral C-spine X-ray
e. **True** – this is to prevent recurrence. The injury causes damage to the posterior ligamentous complex

1.27 Answers

a. **True**
b. **False** – hypotension and bradycardia occur
c. **True**
d. **True**
e. **False** - flexion not extension at the elbow joint

1.28 Answers

a. **True**
b. **True**
c. **False** – need 250 ml of blood present to show globular cardiomegaly
d. **False** – needle pericardiocentesis should only be performed if the patient is peri-arrest
e. **False** – cardiac tamponade is associated with reduced blood pressure, reduced heart sounds, and a raised JVP

1.29 Answers

a. **True**
b. **True**
c. **True**
d. **True**
e. **True**

1.30 Answers

a. **True**
b. **True**
c. **True**
d. **True**
e. **True**

1.31 Answers

a. **False** – nasogastric tube displaces to the right
b. **True**
c. **False** – fracture of upper three ribs
d. **True**
e. **False** – aortic rupture causes upward and rightward shift of the right main stem bronchus

1.32 Answers

a. **True**
b. **True**
c. **True**
d. **True**
e. **False**

1.33 Answers

a. **True**
b. **True**
c. **False**
d. **False**
e. **True**

1.34 Answers

a. **True**
b. **False** – IV cannula should be inserted immediately above the third rib, in the second intercostal space
c. **True**
d. **True**
e. **False** – tension pneumothorax causes tracheal deviation away from the affected side

1.35 Answers

a. **False** – tension pneumothorax causes engorged neck veins due to the restriction of blood flow to the heart
b. **True**
c. **True**
d. **True**
e. **False** – treatment should not be delayed for a CXR

1.36 Answers

a. **True**
b. **True**
c. **True**
d. **True** – as midfacial fracture is a contraindication to intubation
e. **True**

1.37 Answers

a. **False** – jaw thrust manœuvre is contraindicated
b. **False** – false positives may occur with end tidal CO_2 monitoring e.g. after consuming large quantities of carbonated drinks
c. **False** – midfacial fracture is a contraindication to tracheal intubation; cricothyroidotomy should be performed instead
d. **False** – lateral neck X-rays should not be performed if they would delay management
e. **True** – this allows manipulation of their ventilation

1.38 Answers

a. **True**
b. **False** – an ill-fitting blood pressure cuff on the same limb may render readings unreliable
c. **True**
d. **True**
e. **False**

1.39 Answers

a. **True** – due to a relatively blind passage
b. **True** – respirations are needed to help guide correct placement
c. **True**
d. **True**
e. **False**

1.40 Answers

a. **False** – severe respiratory distress is often not obvious
b. **False** – a very painful throat is more indicative of epiglottitis
c. **False** – hypoxia is a late sign of impending obstruction
d. **False** – nebulized adrenaline is recommended for children with moderate-to-severe croup
e. **False** – a 1-day course of prednisolone is usually sufficient

1.41 Answers

a. **True** – due to increased vascularity
b. **False** – associated with an increased risk of pituitary infarction as the pituitary doubles in size during pregnancy
c. **True**
d. **False** – hypoxia occurs faster due to increased needs and decreased functional residual capacity
e. **True** – up to 35% loss may have occurred before any signs occur

1.42 Answers

a. **True**
b. **True** – this is what causes buildings to collapse inwards
c. **False** – secondary blast injuries occur when flying objects strike people
d. **False** – tertiary blast injury is when people fly through the air and strike objects; caused by high energy blasts
e. **True** – to decrease risk of infection

1.43 Answers

a. **True**
b. **True**
c. **False** – > 500 Wbc/mm^3 on DPL
d. **True**
e. **True**

1.44 Answers

a. **True**
b. **True**
c. **True**
d. **False** – stellate wounds are tetanus prone
e. **False** – a depth of > 1 cm is considered to be tetanus prone

1.45 Answers

a. **False** – HATI should be given only if the wound is high-risk; they should all be given a tetanus vaccine however
b. **False**
c. **False**
d. **False** – a course of five vaccinations is considered a complete course
e. **True** – incubation period may be 1 day to 3 months

1.46 Answers

a. **True**
b. **True**
c. **False** – > 50% solution causes immediate tissue destruction
d. **True**
e. **False** – burns are associated with hyperkalaemia as they open calcium-dependent potassium channels in the cell membranes

1.47 Answers

a. **True** – via their effect on calcium-dependent clotting factors
b. **False** – intra-arterial MgSO$_4$ causes tissue necrosis
c. **False** – pain is out of proportion to the physical signs
d. **False**
e. **False** – although it may take up to 24 hours before burns are visible

1.48 Answers

a. **True**
b. **False** – metformin is a contraindication to having an IVU
c. **False** – absence of haematuria may be due to absent kidney, massive parenchymal disruption or renal artery avulsion/thrombosis
d. **True**
e. **False** – myeloma is a contraindication to having an IVU

1.49 Answers

a. **False** – risk of HIV transmission is < 0.3%
b. **False** – 10% risk of hepatitis C transmission versus 30% with hepatitis B
c. **False** – post-exposure prophylaxis should be offered only if a substantial risk is involved
d. **False** – measures to prevent secondary transmission are recommended, especially during the first 6–12 weeks
e. **True**

2. Orthopaedics

2.1 Regarding fractures:

a. Pott's and Weber's classification systems refer to ankle fractures
b. Garden classification system refers to humerus fractures
c. Galeazzi fracture refers to fracture of radial shaft and distal ulna subluxation
d. The metacarpo-phalangeal joint should be splinted in flexion
e. De Quervain's tenosynovitis affects the tendon sheaths of abductor pollicus longus and extensor pollicis brevis

2.2 Regarding fractures:

a. Luxatio erecta refers to posterior shoulder dislocation
b. Maisonneuve fracture refers to fracture of the proximal third of the ulna and radial head subluxation
c. Hill–Sachs lesion refers to avulsion of the joint capsule and glenoid labrum in anterior shoulder dislocation
d. Jefferson fracture refers to an unstable fracture of C1 vertebrae post axial loading
e. A Jones fracture refers to a transverse fracture of the base of fifth metatarsal

2.3 Regarding fracture description:

a. All fractures in children are greenstick fractures
b. Simple fractures refer to fractures with two main fragments
c. Impacted fractures usually involve cancellous bone
d. Sudden contraction of the peroneus brevis may cause fracture at the base of the first metatarsal
e. The lesser trochanter is a common site for avulsion fractures

2.4 Pathological fractures occur in:

a. Paget's disease
b. Osteitis
c. Osteogenesis imperfecta
d. Osteomalacia
e. Fibrosarcoma

2.5   Regarding knee X-rays:

a. Bipartite patella usually affects the inner outer quadrant
b. Abnormal calcification occurs in pseudo gout
c. Osteochondritis dissecans often involves the medial femoral condyle
d. Looser's zones indicate transient growth arrest
e. The fabella represents a loose body

2.6   Increased femoral density on X-ray is associated with:

a. Segmental avascular necrosis
b. Rheumatoid arthritis
c. Osteoarthritis
d. Perthe's disease
e. Osteoporosis

2.7   Regarding cervical spine X-ray:

a. Distance between the arch and the axis is usually 6–7 mm
b. Anterior lipping and disc space narrowing indicate serious trauma
c. A fracture of the spinous process suggests a flexion type injury
d. Calcification of the anterior longitudinal ligament is seen with cervical spondylosis
e. Typically have a convex anterior curvature

2.8   Regarding Salter–Harris classification:

a. Type 1 is a fracture across the growth plate
b. Type 3 involves fracture of the adjacent metaphysis
c. Type 4 is not associated with premature fusion of the growth plate
d. Type 5 is usually easily diagnosed on X-ray
e. Type 5 involves significant misalignment of the bone

2.9   Regarding X-rays:

a. Glass is radio-opaque
b. Patients with suspected biliary disease should have an abdominal X-ray as first-line imaging
c. Ultrasound shows the retrobulbar space better than CT
d. The right heart border is obscured in right lower lobe pneumonia
e. 'Pulled elbow' is most common at age 4–5 years

2.10   Regarding X-rays:

a. The capitate sits in the concavity of the lunate
b. Mallet finger has a bone fragment present in 25% of cases
c. Injuries to the cervical spine are least common in its lower regions
d. Disruption of the symphysis pubis is indicated by a joint space of > 5 mm
e. Hip fractures usually occur anteriorly

2.11 **Regarding X-rays:**

a. The cruciate ligaments of the knee insert into the intercondylar region
b. Calcaneal fractures occur from simple twisting injuries
c. Bohler's angle is increased in calcaneal fractures
d. Avulsion fractures at the base of the fifth metatarsal usually runs longitudinally to the long axis of the metatarsal
e. Acetabulum fractures in association with hip dislocation are rare

2.12 **Carpal tunnel syndrome associations:**

a. Rheumatoid arthritis
b. Hypothyroidism
c. Addison's disease
d. Diabetes mellitus
e. Hyperparathyroidism

2.13 **Regarding shoulder joint pathology:**

a. Rotator cuff tears most commonly involve the supraspinatus region
b. Rotator cuff tears usually require a large force to occur
c. There is an increased incidence of frozen shoulder after a Colles' fracture
d. Osteoarthritis is more common than rheumatoid arthritis
e. Rotator cuff is composed of supraspinatus, infraspinatus, subscapularis, and teres major

2.14 **Causes of foot pain:**

a. Plantar neuroma
b. Freiberg's disease
c. Kohler's disease
d. Ankylosing spondylitis
e. Posterior tibial nerve compression

2.15 **Regarding leg pain:**

a. Tibial osteitis causes tenderness of the diaphyseal area
b. Spinal stenosis causes leg pain
c. Shin splints and stress fractures may be confused
d. The tibia is a rare site for primary bone tumours in children
e. Osteitis of the tibia may cause an inability to weight bear

2.16 **Regarding knee pathology:**

a. Osgood–Schlatter's disease usually resolves with closure of the epiphysis
b. Osgood–Schlatter's disease usually affects 7–10 year olds
c. A torn meniscus causes a haemarthrosis
d. The patella has a tendency to dislocate medially
e. Anterior cruciate ligament tears are often associated with medial meniscus tears

2.17 Regarding knee pathology:

a. Locking of the knee occurs in full extension
b. Osteoarthritis affects the medial compartment first
c. Chondromalacia patella usually affects females between the ages of 15 and 35 years
d. Genu varum (bow leg) occurs in Paget's disease
e. Dashboard injuries may tear the posterior cruciate ligament

2.18 Regarding hand pathology:

a. Dupuytren's contracture is associated with thickening of the plantar fascia
b. Dupuytren's contracture occurs most commonly in females
c. Mallet finger is caused by rupture of the flexor digitorum profundus
d. Boutonniere deformity is caused by detachment of the central slip of the extensor tendon
e. Trigger finger is most common in the middle and ring finger

2.19 Regarding wrist joint pathology:

a. Ulnar nerve passes between the pisiform and hook of hamate
b. There are 10 carpal bones
c. Ganglions are associated with neurological complications
d. Carpal tunnel syndrome is more common in males
e. Ulnar tunnel syndrome affects both the sensory and motor divisions of the ulnar nerve

2.20 Regarding hip joint pathology:

a. Most common cause of hip pain in an adult is referred pain from the spine
b. Psoas spasm may cause a flexion contraction
c. After hip replacement, component loosening may be caused by infection
d. Fractures of the femoral neck may occur without a history of trauma
e. Shenton's lines on X-ray run from the inferior pubic ramus to the femoral neck

2.21 Regarding cervical rib syndrome:

a. It involves the brachial plexus and axillary artery
b. Causes hypothenar and not thenar wasting
c. Often causes pain along the ulnar border of the hand
d. Is associated with gangrene
e. Usually is associated with bilateral symptoms of ischaemia

2.22 Regarding elbow joint pathology:

    a. Pain in the region of the medial epicondyle indicates golfer's elbow
    b. Pulled elbow in children causes loss of supination only
    c. Myositis ossificans causes a mechanical block to extension
    d. Lack of physiotherapy after injury predisposes to myositis ossificans
    e. Aspiration is typically done from the medial aspect of the elbow joint

2.23 Regarding hip injuries:

    a. Intracapsular fractures are more common than extracapsular
    b. The Garden classification system describes extracapsular neck of femur fractures
    c. Neck of femur fractures cause adduction and internal rotation of the lower limb
    d. Dislocation is usually in an anterior direction
    e. Femoral head avascular necrosis is a complication of extracapsular femoral neck fracture

2.24 Regarding brachial plexus injuries:

    a. Motorcycle accidents are the most common cause
    b. Damage to the nerve to the serratus anterior causes winging of the scapula
    c. Bruising in the posterior triangle carries a poor prognosis
    d. Fracture of a transverse process has a poor prognosis
    e. Suprascapular nerve arises from the lower trunk

2.25 Regarding upper brachial plexus injury:

    a. Causes loss of supination
    b. Causes loss of flexion at metacarpal phalangeal joints
    c. Causes loss of lateral upper arm sensation
    d. Causes loss of extension at the interphalangeal joints
    e. Causes loss of abduction and external rotation of the shoulder joint

2.26 Regarding lower brachial plexus injury:

    a. Causes claw hand
    b. Causes loss of biceps function
    c. Apical lung carcinoma may cause this
    d. Is associated with ptosis
    e. Causes Erb's palsy

2.27 Regarding Colles' fracture:

a. Is associated with delayed rupture of extensor pollicis brevis
b. Is associated with carpal tunnel syndrome
c. Bilateral fractures should be manipulated with a Bier's blockade
d. Is associated with anterior displacement of the distal radial fragment
e. Is associated with scaphoid fractures

2.28 Regarding scaphoid fractures:

a. Majority occur at the proximal pole
b. Avascular necrosis is common with fractures of the distal pole
c. There is an increased incidence of rheumatoid arthritis after a fracture
d. A fracture of the tuberosity requires POP fixation
e. Is associated with proximal ulna fractures

2.29 Regarding supracondylar fractures in children:

a. Complications include myositis ossificans
b. 5% lateral angulation is an indication for fixation
c. > 50% displacement is an indication for fixation
d. Median nerve injury is associated
e. Neurovascular compromise is not an indication for fixation

2.30 Regarding elbow joint dislocations:

a. Most common neurovascular complication involves the median nerve
b. This is one of the most common joint dislocations
c. Usually dislocates posterolaterally
d. After reduction the joint should be immobilized in a cylinder cast
e. Patient typically presents holding the forearm extended

2.31 Regarding foot fractures:

a. LisFranc injuries refer to metatarsal fractures
b. Lateral side of the second metatarsal should be aligned with the medial side of the middle cuneiform
c. Dislocated metatarsals are an orthopaedic emergency
d. Most common site for stress fractures is the second metatarsal
e. Displaced talar fractures have a high incidence of avascular necrosis

2.32 Regarding nerve root lesions:

a. Absent ankle reflex, poor foot plantar flexion, and intact knee flexion: S1, S2 lesion
b. Absent supinator reflex, poor elbow flexion, and intact triceps reflex: C6 lesion
c. Absent knee reflex, poor knee extension, and poor foot dorsiflexion: L5, S1 lesion
d. Absent biceps reflex and poor shoulder abduction: C6 lesion
e. Limb weakness and sacral sensation sparing: intermedullary lesion

2.33 The following fractures and nerve injuries are associated:

a. Proximal fibular fracture and weak ankle plantar flexion
b. Posterior shoulder dislocation and deltoid weakness
c. Lunate dislocation and ulnar nerve injury
d. Posterior hip dislocation and weak ankle dorsiflexion
e. Supracondylar fracture and loss of sensation of the little finger

2.34 The following nerve injuries and reflexes are associated:

a. C5 – loss of biceps jerk
b. C6 – loss of wrist flexion
c. C6 – loss of pronation
d. S1 – loss of ankle dorsiflexion
e. L4 – loss of knee extension

2.35 Regarding the radial nerve:

a. Colles' fracture is a common cause of impairment
b. Crutches can cause a radial nerve palsy
c. Wasting of the triceps is a sign of palsy
d. Facilitates pronation of the forearm
e. Is derived from the anterior cord of the brachial plexus

2.36 Regarding radial nerve injuries:

a. Common cause of injury is fracture of the midshaft humerus
b. Causes wrist drop
c. Causes loss of extension of the elbow joint
d. Causes loss of sensation over the first palmer interosseous muscle
e. Causes loss of triceps function

2.37 Median nerve injury at the elbow joint:

a. Causes loss of adductor pollicis
b. Causes loss of supinator
c. Causes loss of thumb opposition
d. Causes sensory loss of the radial four and a half digits
e. May be caused by supracondylar fracture or a tight bicipital aponeurosis

2.38   Regarding ulnar nerve injury:

a. Injury at the wrist causes loss of flexor carpi ulnaris and flexor digitorum profundus
b. Injury at wrist causes loss of all the intrinsic muscles of the hand
c. Injury at the elbow causes sensory loss to the little finger
d. Injury at the elbow joint causes clawing of the hand
e. Often caused by damage to the lateral epicondyle

2.39   Regarding radial nerve damage at the wrist joint:

a. Causes loss of thumb opposition and abduction
b. Causes loss of thumb flexion
c. Causes loss of adductor pollicis
d. Causes 'ape-like' hand
e. Causes Benediction attitude in the hand

2.40   Regarding Sudeck's atrophy:

a. Colles' fracture is the most common type of fracture to cause this
b. Sympathetic blockade is of diagnostic value
c. Osteoporotic bony changes are seen on X-ray
d. Only occurs post fractures
e. Only affects the upper limbs

2.41   Regarding Sudeck's atrophy:

a. Is associated with osteodystrophy
b. Is associated with hyper-reflexia
c. Is associated with joint space narrowing on X-ray
d. Chemical sympathectomy is commonly used in management
e. Intensive physiotherapy should be avoided

2.42   Increased risk of avascular necrosis is associated with:

a. Alcohol abuse
b. Diabetes
c. Severe osteoarthritis
d. Sever's disease
e. Gaucher's disease

2.43   Compartment syndrome:

a. Crush injury is a common cause
b. Pain increases with passive muscle stretch
c. Compartment pressure is > 35–45 mmHg
d. Loss of pedal pulses is an early sign in lower leg compartment syndrome
e. May be caused by tibial osteitis

2.44   Anterior tibial compartment syndrome:

   a. Extensor hallucis longus is commonly the first muscle affected
   b. The deep peroneal nerve is affected
   c. Causes an absent posterior tibial pulse
   d. Causes an absent dorsalis pedis pulse
   e. Causes weak ankle and great toe extension

2.45   Regarding temperomandibular joint dislocation:

   a. Unilateral dislocation is more common than bilateral
   b. It causes earache and inability to fully close the jaw
   c. The condyle is usually anteriorly dislocated
   d. If unilateral the jaw deviates to the unaffected side
   e. Risk of cartilage damage mandates maxillofacial follow-up

2.46   Regarding hip pathology in children:

   a. Typical age of onset for Perthes' disease is 3–10 years old
   b. Sclerosis and an increased lateral joint space are seen on X-ray
      in patients with Perthes' disease
   c. Slipped upper femoral epiphysis is more common in males
   d. All children with hip pain should have a plain X-ray of the
      affected hip
   e. Slipped upper femoral epiphysis is usually conservatively
      managed

2.47   Regarding eponymous osteochondritis:

   a. Kienbock's disease is an osteochondritis of the lunate
   b. Freiberg's disease is an osteochondritis of the naviculum
   c. Sever's, Sinding–Larsen's and Osgood–Schlatter's are all types
      of traction apophysitis
   d. Kohler's disease is an osteochondritis of the capitate
   e. Scheuermann's disease is an osteochondritis of the vertebrae

2.48   Regarding osteosarcomas:

   a. They affect the diaphysis of bones
   b. Commonly occur at the distal humerus
   c. Pain is usually worse post exercise
   d. Associated with Codman's triangle
   e. Associated with retinoblastoma

2.49   Causes of foot drop:

   a. Motor neuron disease
   b. Sciatic nerve injury
   c. Thyrotoxicosis
   d. Common peroneal nerve injury
   e. S1 nerve root injury

2.50 **Regarding osteomyelitis:**

a. Affects bone growth
b. Fractures cause increased susceptibility
c. Most common pathogen is *Staph. aureus*
d. Usually the metaphysis is first affected
e. Associated with Brodie's abscess

2.51 **Regarding fractures and child abuse:**

a. Ribs and humerus are common sites
b. Average case has three to four fractures
c. Growth plate injuries are common
d. Skull X-ray may show widening of the sutures
e. Fractures with a vague history require further investigation

2.1 Answers

a. **True**
b. **False** – Garden classification system refers to hip fractures
c. **True**
d. **True**
e. **True**

2.2 Answers

a. **False** – luxato erecta refers to inferior shoulder dislocation
b. **False** – fracture of the proximal third of the ulna and radial head subluxation describes a Monteggia fracture. A Maisonneuve injury is an unstable injury with rupture of the medial ankle ligament and proximal fibula fracture
c. **False** – avulsion of the joint capsule and glenoid labrum is a Bankart lesion. A Hill–Sachs lesion is an impacted compression of the humeral head which occurs during anterior shoulder dislocation
d. **True**
e. **True**

2.3 Answers

a. **False** – although greenstick fractures occur in children, not all fractures are greenstick
b. **True**
c. **True**
d. **False** – sudden contraction of the peroneus ~~brevis~~ *longus* causes fractures at base of fifth metatarsal
e. **True** – due to sudden forceful contraction of the iliopsoas muscle

2.4 Answers

a. **True** – usually affecting the tibia and femur
b. **True**
c. **True**
d. **True**
e. **True**

2.5 Answers

a. **False** – bipartite patella usually affects the upper outer quadrant
b. **True**
c. **True**
d. **True**
e. **False** – the fabella is a sesmoid bone

2.6 Answers

a. **True**
b. **False** – rheumatoid arthritis is associated with reduced density
c. **False**
d. **True**
e. **False** – osteoporosis is associated with reduced density

2.7 Answers

a. **False** – 1–4 mm. The distance is increased in rupture or laxity of the transverse ligament, e.g. in trauma, infection, or rheumatoid arthritis

b. **False** – anterior lipping and disc space narrowing are typical findings in cervical spondylosis

c. **True**

d. **False** – calcification of the anterior longitudinal ligament is seen with ankylosing spondylitis; widespread fusion of the facet joints is also seen

e. **True**

2.8 Answers

a. **True**

b. **False** – the epiphysis only is affected in Type 3

c. **False**

d. **False** – Type 5 is often difficult to see on plain X-ray as it is an impaction fracture of the entire growth plate

e. **False**

2.9 Answers

a. **True**

b. **False** – ultrasound is the imaging modality of choice in patients with suspected biliary disease

c. **False** – CT is superior to ultrasound in showing the retrobulbar space

d. **False** – the right heart border is obscured in right middle lobe pneumonia

e. **False** – 'pulled elbow' is usually outgrown by age 4–5 years

2.10 Answers

a. **True**

b. **True**

c. **False** – the C5–C7 region is the most commonly affected

d. **True**

e. **False** – 80% of hip fractures are posterior

2.11 Answers

a. **True**

b. **True** – although rare, calcaneal fractures may occur. Most common after a fall from a height

c. **False** – Bohler's angle is reduced to < 30 degrees in calcaneal fractures. Normal angle is between 30 and 40 degrees

d. **False** – This suggests an apophysis. Fractures usually run transverse to the long axis

e. **False** – acetabulum fractures are commonly associated with hip dislocation

2.12 Answers

a. **True**
b. **True**
c. **False**
d. **True**
e. **False**

2.13 Answers

a. **True**
b. **False** – in the elderly, rupture often occurs spontaneously
c. **True** – increased incidence of frozen shoulder is seen after prolonged arm rest from any cause
d. **False**
e. **False** – the teres minor not the teres major is part of the rotator cuff

2.14 Answers

a. **True** – plantar neuroma occurs at the bifurcation of the nerve at the toe cleft
b. **True** – Frieberg's disease is an osteochondritis of the second metatarsal head
c. **True** – Kohler's disease is an osteochondritis of the naviculum
d. **False** – ankylosing spondylitis is a cause of knee and hip pain
e. **True** – posterior tibial nerve compression is tarsal tunnel syndrome

2.15 Answers

a. **False** – tibial osteitis causes tenderness of the metaphyseal area
b. **True**
c. **True** – both shin splints and stress fractures cause tenderness along the posteromedial border
d. **False** – the tibia is a common site for primary bone tumours in children
e. **True**

2.16 Answers

a. **True**
b. **False** – Osgood–Schlatter's disease usually affects 10–16 year olds
c. **False** – The meniscus is avascular. If it becomes detached at the periphery it may cause a haemarthrosis
d. **False** – the patella has a tendency to dislocate laterally
e. **True**

2.17 Answers

a. **False** – locking of the knee never occurs in full extension.
b. **True**
c. **True** – chondromalacia patella is caused by softening of the articular cartilage lining the patella
d. **True**
e. **True**

2.18 Answers

a. **True**
b. **False** – Dupuytren's contracture is more common in males
c. **False** – Mallet finger is caused by rupture of the distal slip of the extensor tendon
d. **True** – at its attachment to the base of the middle phalanx
e. **True**

2.19 Answers

a. **True**
b. **False** – there are eight: capitate, scaphoid, hamate, lunate, pisiform, trapezium, trapezoid, triquetral
c. **True** – if ganglions are in close proximity to peripheral nerves
d. **False** – carpal tunnel syndrome is more common in females
e. **True** – although often only one of the divisions of the ulnar nerve is affected

2.20 Answers

a. **True** – most often from a prolapsed intervertebral disc
b. **True** – due to inflammation in the region of the sheath in the pelvis
c. **True**
d. **True**
e. **False** – Shenton's lines run from the superior pubic ramus to the femoral neck

2.21 Answers

a. **True**
b. **False** – cervical rib syndrome usually causes wasting of both the thenar and hypothenar muscles
c. **True**
d. **True** – gangrene of the fingertips if there is complete vascular occlusion
e. **False** – cervical rib syndrome is usually associated unilateral symptoms of ischaemia. Bilateral symptoms are more common in Raynaud's disease

2.22 Answers

a. **True**
b. **True**
c. **False** – myositis ossificans causes a mechanical block to flexion
d. **False** – myositis ossificans is more common after overactive physiotherapy
e. **False** – aspiration is usually done from the lateral aspect to avoid the ulnar nerve

2.23 Answers

a. **False** – extracapsular fractures are four times more common than intracapsular fractures
b. **False** – the Garden classification system describes intracapsular neck of femur fractures
c. **False** – neck of femur fracture causes the lower limb to be held in external rotation and abduction
d. **False** – 85–90% of cases dislocate posteriorly
e. **False** – it is a complication of intracapsular neck of femur fractures

2.24 Answers

a. **True**
b. **True**
c. **True** – bruising indicates a preganglionic lesion and injury to the roots of the brachial plexus
d. **True**
e. **False** – supracapsular nerve arises from the upper trunk – C5, C6; supplies supraspinatus and infraspinatus

2.25 Answers

a. **True**
b. **False** – lower brachial plexus injuries cause loss of flexion at metacarpal phalangeal joints
c. **True**
d. **False** – loss of extension at the interphalangeal joints is associated with lower brachial plexus injuries
e. **True** – due to loss of the deltoid and short shoulder muscles

2.26 Answers

a. **True**
b. **False** – upper brachial plexus injuries cause loss of biceps function
c. **True**
d. **True** – if there is damage to the sympathetic chain
e. **False** – Erb's palsy is associated with upper brachial plexus injuries

2.27 Answers

a. **False** – Colles' fracture is associated with delayed rupture of extensor pollicis longus
b. **True**
c. **False** – bilateral fractures are a contraindication to Bier's blockade
d. **False** – Colles' fracture is associated with posterior displacement of the distal radial fragment
e. **True** – scaphoid fractures are often missed in patients with a Colles' fracture

2.28 Answers

a. **False** – 50% of scaphoid fractures occur at the waist and approximately 38% at the proximal pole
b. **False** – avascular necrosis is more common with proximal pole fractures
c. **False** – There is increased incidence of osteoarthritis after a fracture
d. **False** – POP fixation is not required as avascular necrosis does not occur with tuberosity fractures
e. **False** – scaphoid fractures are associated with distal ulna fractures

2.29 Answers

a. **True**
b. **False** – 10% lateral angulation is an indication for fixation
c. **True**
d. **True**
e. **False**

2.30 Answers

a. **False** – most common neurovascular complication involves the ulnar nerve
False b. ~~**True**~~ – elbow joint dislocation is the third most common joint dislocation after glenohumeral and patello femoral dislocations
c. **True**
d. **False** – the joint should not be immobilized in a cylinder cast due to the likely risk of a large amount of soft tissue swelling
e. **False** – typically the forearm is held at a 45-degree angle to the body

2.31 Answers

a. **False** – Lisfranc injuries refer to tarso–metatarsal dislocation
b. **False** – the medial side of the second metatarsal should be aligned with the medial side of the middle cuneiform
c. **True**
d. **True**
e. **True**

2.32 Answers

a. **True**
b. **True**
c. **False** – L3, L4 lesion
d. **False** – C5 lesion
e. **True** – intermedullary lesion spares the lateral spinothalamic tracts which causes sparing of sacral sensation

2.33 Answers

a. **False** – weak ankle dorsiflexion via the common peroneal nerve
b. **True** – via the axillary nerve
c. **False** – lunate dislocation is associated with median nerve injury
d. **True** – via the sciatic nerve
e. **False** – supracondylar fracture is associated with median nerve injury and hence loss of index finger sensation

2.34 Answers

a. **True**
b. **True**
c. **True**
d. **False** – L4, L5 innervation
e. **False** – L3 innervation

2.35 Answers

a. **False** – Colles' fracture is associated with median nerve palsy
b. **True** – from pressure on the nerve in the axilla
c. **True**
d. **False** – radial nerve supplies the forearm supinator
e. **False** – radial nerve is derived from the posterior cord

2.36 Answers

a. **True**
b. **True**
c. **False** – radial nerve injuries cause loss of extension of the wrist joint
d. **False** – radial nerve injuries cause loss of sensation over the first dorsal interosseous muscle
e. **False**

2.37 Answers

a. **False** – median nerve injury at the elbow joint causes the loss of the remaining thenar muscles
b. **False** – median nerve injury at the elbow joint causes loss of pronator teres
c. **True**
d. **False** – median nerve injury at the elbow joint causes sensory loss of the radial three and a half digits
e. **True**

2.38 Answers

a. **False** – loss of flexor digitorum profundus indicates an ulnar nerve lesion at or near the elbow joint
b. **False** – ulnar nerve injury at the wrist does not affect the two radial lumbricals
c. **True**
d. **True**
e. **False** – damage to the medial epicondyle may cause ulnar nerve damage

2.39 Answers

a. **True**
b. **False** – the flexor pollicis longus is unaffected
c. **False** – the other thenar muscles are affected however
d. **True** – due to loss of function of the thenar muscles
e. **False** – Benediction attitude is seen in radial nerve injuries at the elbow joint; damage at the wrist joint leaves the long flexor muscles intact

2.40 Answers

a. **True**
b. **True** – sympathetic blockade is diagnostic if it causes pain relief for 1–4 days post infusion
c. **True**
d. **False** – Sudeck's atrophy can occur after seemingly minor soft tissue injuries
e. **False** – Sudeck's atrophy can also affect the lower limbs

2.41 Answers

a. **False**
b. **True**
c. **False** – Sudeck's atrophy is associated with widening of the joint space
d. **False** – chemical sympathectomy is rarely used
e. **False** – intensive physiotherapy is recommended in management

2.42 Answers

a. **True**
b. **True**
c. **True**
d. **False** – Sever's disease is an Achilles tendon traction injury which causes chronic heel pain in children
e. **True**

2.43 Answers

a. **True**
b. **True**
c. **True**
d. **False** – loss of pedal pulses is a late sign in lower leg compartment syndrome
e. **False**

2.44 Answers

a. **True** – along with the tibialis anterior
b. **True**
c. **False**
d. **True**
e. **True**

2.45 Answers

a. **False** – bilateral dislocation is more common
b. **True**
c. **True**
d. **False** – the jaw deviates to the affected side
e. **True**

2.46 Answers

a. **True**
b. **False** – sclerosis and an increased medial joint space are seen on X-ray
c. **True**
d. **False** – hip ultrasound is often the sole imaging modality required
e. **False** – surgical fixation to minimize risk of avascular necrosis is often employed

2.47 Answers

a. **True**
b. **False** – Freiberg's disease is an osteochondritis of the second metatarsal head
c. **True**
d. **False** – Kohler's disease is an osteochondritis of the naviculum
e. **True**

2.48 Answers

a. **False** – osteosarcomas affect the metaphyseal region of bones
b. **False** – the proximal humerus is a common site for osteosarcomas
c. **True**
d. **True** – Codman's triangle is a sign of periosteal elevation
e. **True** – in Li Fraumeni syndrome

2.49 Answers

a. **True**
b. **True**
c. **False**
d. **True**
e. **False** – L4, L5 nerve root lesion

2.50 Answers

a. **True** – if the epiphysis is involved
b. **True** – if compound fracture
c. **True** – in all age groups
d. **True**
e. **True** – Brodie's abscess is a bone abscess indicating subacute infection

2.51 Answers

a. **True**
b. **True**
c. **False** – growth plate injuries are usually caused by other forms of trauma
d. **True**
e. **True**

3. Medical

3.1 Pulse associations:

a. Pulsus alternans and left ventricular failure
b. Pulsus paradoxus and COPD
c. Plateau pulse and aortic regurgitation
d. Pulsus bisferiens and mixed aortic stenosis and incompetence
e. Pulsus paradoxus and cardiac tamponade

3.2 Regarding heart sounds:

a. S4 occurs in aortic stenosis
b. S3 is associated with aortic regurgitation
c. Right-sided heart murmurs are loudest during inspiration
d. Third heart sound is always pathological
e. Fourth heart sound is caused by reduced compliance of the left ventricle

3.3 ECG associations:

a. WPW and reduced PR interval
b. Hyperkalaemia and peaked T waves
c. Hypercalcaemia and prolonged QT interval
d. Ischaemia and inverted T waves
e. Hypocalcaemia and prolonged QT interval

3.4 Regarding sympathetic nerve supply:

a. Predominately vasoconstrictor
b. Causes pupillary constriction
c. Causes tremor
d. Causes tachycardia
e. Causes sweating

3.5 Clubbing associations:

a. Thyrotoxicosis
b. Small cell lung carcinoma
c. Empyema
d. Whipple's disease
e. Diverticulosis

3.6 **Regarding mitral stenosis:**

a. Associated with a prominent A wave in central venous pressure readings
b. Associated with loss of A wave in central venous pressure readings
c. Associated with an opening snap
d. Associated with a tapping heart sound
e. Associated with a systolic murmur

3.7 **Aortic regurgitation associations:**

a. Dissecting aneurysm
b. Marfan's disease
c. Ankylosing spondylitis
d. Thyrotoxicosis
e. Raynaud's disease

3.8 **Regarding aortic regurgitation associations:**

a. Hill's sign
b. Opening snap
c. Wide pulse pressure
d. Quincke's sign
e. Phalen's sign

3.9 **Regarding aortic stenosis associations:**

a. Plateau pulse
b. S4
c. Hyperdynamic apex beat
d. Diastolic murmur at the left sternal edge
e. Mid systolic ejection murmur at the aortic area

3.10 **Causes of a dominant A wave in CVP readings:**

a. Pulmonary hypertension
b. Pulmonary stenosis
c. Tricuspid stenosis
d. Complete heart block
e. Tricuspid regurgitation

3.11 **Increased resonance is found with the following:**

a. Mesothelioma
b. Acute asthma
c. Pneumothorax
d. Small cell lung carcinoma
e. Hyperventilation

3.12 Pericarditis associations:

a. Systemic lupus erythematosis
b. Hydralazine
c. Q waves on ECG
d. Convex upward ST segments
e. Antibiotic treatment in all cases

3.13 Regarding myocardial infarction:

a. Posterior myocardial infarction is associated with concave upwards ST depression
b. Right-sided myocardial infarction usually occurs as part of an inferior myocardial infarction
c. Subendocardial myocardial infarction is associated with ST elevation
d. Right ventricular failure usually requires diuretics
e. Right-sided myocardial infarction causes ST elevation in V1

3.14 The following cause a prolonged QT interval:

a. Hypocalcaemia
b. Digoxin
c. Sleep
d. Hyperthermia
e. Imipramine

3.15 Regarding central venous pressure waves:

a. A wave = atrial contraction
b. C wave = atrial filling with a closed tricuspid valve
c. Large A waves occur in atrial fibrillation
d. X descent = atrial relaxation
e. Giant V waves occur in tricuspid regurgitation

3.16 Regarding nitroglycerin:

a. Contraindicated in right ventricular infarction
b. Contraindicated if the systolic blood pressure is < 90 mmHg
c. Should never be used for > 48 hours
d. Aim for a > 30% blood pressure drop if hypertensive
e. Is light sensitive

3.17 Regarding ACE inhibitors:

a. Improve left ventricular dysfunction in patients after an acute myocardial infarction
b. Decrease sudden death post myocardial infarction
c. Contraindicated if left ventricular ejection fraction is < 40%
d. Contraindicated in pregnancy
e. Increased doses are needed if in renal failure

3.18 Regarding beta-blockers:

a. Decrease the incidence of ventricular fibrillation post acute myocardial infarction
b. Cause reduced myocardial ischaemia in patients with left ventricular dysfunction
c. Used as a first-line agent to control tachyarrhythmias
d. Contraindicated if systolic blood pressure is < 120 mmHg
e. Contraindicated in second- or third-degree heart block

3.19 Drugs that prolong the QT interval:

a. Amiodarone
b. Procainamide
c. Co-amoxiclav
d. Sotalol
e. Flucloxacillin

3.20 Regarding calcium channel blockers:

a. Cause hypotension
b. Indicated in patients with left ventricular dysfunction
c. Useful to terminate PSVT with narrow QRS complexes
d. Useful in atrial fibrillation and WPW
e. Avoid if in third-degree heart block without a pacemaker in situ

3.21 Regarding WPW:

a. Calcium channel blockers are used in its management
b. Associated with U waves
c. Associated with a short PR interval
d. Associated with mitral valve prolapse
e. Associated with a dominant R wave in V1

3.22 The following cause raised digoxin levels:

a. Verapamil
b. Hypoxia
c. Quinine
d. Hypercalcaemia
e. Hypothyroidism

3.23 Regarding atrial flutter:

a. Associated with hyperthyroidism
b. Carotid sinus pressure helps to reveal flutter waves
c. There are often more A waves present in the CVP than are palpable in the pulse
d. Associated with a heart rate of 150 bpm
e. Sotalol is contraindicated due to high risk of causing ventricular tachycardia

3.24 Regarding atrial fibrillation:

a. Sotalol is recommended for rate control
b. Associated with hypothermia
c. Adenosine is used in treatment
d. Associated with fusion beats on an ECG
e. Calcium chloride is used in treatment

3.25 Causes of heart block:

a. Inferior myocardial infarction
b. Digoxin toxicity
c. Sick sinus syndrome
d. Aortic valve disease
e. Gullain–Barré syndrome

3.26 Ventricular tachyarrhythmia associations:

a. Cannon A waves
b. QRS complexes > 140 ms
c. Atrioventicular dissociation
d. Capture beats
e. Dilated cardiomyopathy

3.27 Ventricular tachyarrhythmia adverse symptoms:

a. Loss of consciousness
b. Pulselessness
c. Systolic blood pressure < 90 mmHg
d. Chest pain
e. Heart rate > 120 bpm

3.28 Bradycardia associations:

a. Adenosine is used in management
b. Increased risk of asytole with complete heart block
c. May cause complete heart block
d. Adverse signs include systolic blood pressure < 90 mmHg
e. Adverse signs include heart rate < 40 bpm

3.29 Regarding broad complex tachycardia:

a. All patients with torsades de pointes should receive defibrillation
b. Verapamil is used in management
c. Class 1 anti-arrhythmics may cause ventricular tachycardia
d. IV amiodarone is used in management
e. Tricyclic antidepressants and phenothiazine may cause ventricular tachycardia

3.30 Regarding cardiogenic pulmonary oedema:

a. Associated with raised JVP
b. Associated with a third and fourth heart sound
c. IV opioid use is contraindicated
d. If PaO_2 < 9 kPa, ventilatory support is recommended
e. If hypotensive, fluid resuscitation is recommended

3.31 Regarding infective endocarditis:

a. Associated with splenomegaly
b. Associated with renal dysfunction
c. *Staph. aureus* causes more neurological side-effects than *Strep. viridans*
d. All patients should receive anticoagulation
e. Coexistent congestive cardiac failure is a poor prognostic factor

3.32 Causes of hypotension with a raised JVP include:

a. Acute severe asthma
b. Ruptured aortic aneurysm
c. Uraemia
d. Splenic tamponade
e. Biventricular failure

3.33 Regarding angina:

a. Mild left ventricular failure is a contraindication to beta-blockade
b. Thrombolytic agents are useful in unstable angina
c. Tolerance may occur to IV GTN
d. Potassium channel openers may be used in refractory angina
e. Calcium antagonists do not decrease the risk of myocardial infarction in patients with unstable angina

3.34 Causes of atrial fibrillation:

a. Pulmonary embolus
b. Hypertension
c. Hypokalaemia
d. Empyema
e. Hypomagnesaesia

3.35 Indications for beta-blockade post myocardial infarction:

a. AV block
b. Recurrent ischaemic pain
c. Left ventricular failure
d. Hyperdynamic state
e. SBP < 95 mmHg

3.36 Thrombolysis is particularly useful for patients with:

a. Anterior infarcts
b. Patients older than 75 years
c. Ulcerative colitis and acute myocardial infarction
d. Renal disease and acute myocardial infarction
e. SBP < 100 mmHg

3.37 Myocardial infarction complications:

a. Fever
b. Mitral regurgitation
c. Ventricular septal defect
d. Ventricular ectopics
e. Ruptured papillary muscle

3.38 Regarding dysrhythmias post myocardial infarction:

a. Inferior myocardial infarction is associated with sinus bradycardia
b. Anterior myocardial infarction is associated with third-degree heart block
c. Ventricular ectopics are treated with $MgSO_4$
d. All episodes of bradycardia should be treated
e. Ventricular ectopics post myocardial infarction have a poor long-term prognosis

3.39 Severe asthma indicators:

a. Restricted daily activities
b. Peripheral cyanosis
c. Difficulty in speaking
d. Pulse rate of 110 bpm
e. Peak expiratory flow rate of 70% of predicted value

3.40 Regarding pulmonary embolus:

a. High-risk patients should have D-dimer test performed
b. Intermediate-risk patients should all have a CTPA
c. Isotope lung scanning is not recommended in a patient with COPD
d. Is associated with right ventricular gallop
e. Is associated with T inversion in V1, V2, and right axis deviation on ECG

3.41 Regarding asthma:

a. Immediate treatment of acute severe asthma includes sedatives for anxiety
b. All patients require a CXR
c. Patients with deteriorating PEF despite optimum management require ITU
d. IV $MgSO_4$ is indicated if life-threatening features are present
e. IV aminophylline is contraindicated in acute severe asthma

3.42 **The following are features of life-threatening asthma:**

a. $SpO_2 < 92\%$
b. $PaCO_2 < 4.6$ kPa
c. $PaO_2 < 8$ kPa
d. Inability to complete full sentences
e. PEF 33–50% of normal expected value

3.43 **Pneumothorax:**

a. Is associated with Marfan's syndrome
b. Is associated with cocaine
c. ECG signs include reduced QRS amplitude and T inversion in praecordial leads
d. Aspiration is deemed successful if excessive coughing is stimulated
e. Tetracycline and talc are used for pleurodesis

3.44 **Pneumothorax:**

a. Over 50% recur in the first 4 years post pneumothorax
b. Secondary pneumothorax has milder symptoms than primary pneumothorax
c. All patients should receive high flow oxygen
d. Risk associated with diving returns to baseline normal after 6 months
e. Post successful aspiration patients with a secondary pneumothorax can be safely discharged

3.45 **Pneumonia:**

a. *Staph. aureus* is associated with cavitating lesions on CXR
b. *Haem. influenzae* is the most common bacterial cause
c. $PaO_2 < 10$ kpa is a poor prognostic indicator
d. Urea of 14 is a poor prognostic indicator
e. Respiratory rate of > 30 is a poor prognostic indicator

3.46 **Regarding the ABG: pH 7.22, $PaCO_2$ 55, HCO_3 25:**

a. Shows a respiratory acidosis
b. Shows a metabolic acidosis
c. Consistent with pyloric stenosis
d. Consistent with COPD

3.47 **Regarding the ABG: pH 7.50, $PaCO_2$ 42, HCO_3 33:**

a. Shows a metabolic alkalosis
b. Intravenous fluids may help normalize this patients ABGs
c. Consistent with COPD
d. Consistent with a patient with gastroenteritis

3.48 Regarding the ABG: pH 7.35, $PaCO_2$ 48, HCO_3 28:

   a. Consistent with COPD
   b. Consistent with a morbidly obese patient
   c. Consistent with a patient with an acute exacerbation of asthma
   d. Consistent with a patient with chronic diaphragmatic paralysis

3.49 Regarding the ABG: pH 7.32, $PaCO_2$ 32, HCO_3 18:

   a. Shows a metabolic acidosis
   b. Shows a metabolic alkalosis
   c. Consistent with a vomiting patient
   d. Shows a respiratory acidosis

3.50 The following show a partially compensated respiratory acidosis:

   a. pH 7.43, $PaCO_2$ 48, HCO_3 36
   b. pH 7.33, $PaCO_2$ 62, HCO_3 35
   c. pH 7.33, $PaCO_2$ 62, HCO_3 28
   d. pH 7.5, $PaCO_2$ 43, HCO_3 36

3.51 Adult respiratory distress syndrome is associated with:

   a. Septicaemia
   b. Raised intracranial pressure
   c. Salicylate overdose
   d. Burns
   e. Deep vein thrombosis

3.52 Causes of hyperkalaemia:

   a. Metabolic acidosis
   b. Pyloric stenosis
   c. Spironolactone
   d. Addison's disease
   e. Excess liquorice intake

3.53 Hyperkalaemia ECG changes:

   a. Wide QRS complex
   b. Sine wave rhythm
   c. Peaked T waves
   d. Delta waves
   e. U waves

3.54 Causes of SIADH:

   a. Opiates
   b. Cerebrovascular accident
   c. Subarachnoid haemorrhage
   d. Prostate cancer
   e. Trauma

3.55 Hyponatraemia associations:

a. Addison's disease
b. Liver cirrhosis
c. Trauma
d. Diabetes insipidus
e. Primary hyperaldosteronism

3.56 Hypercalcaemia is associated with:

a. Tetany
b. Trousseau's sign
c. Acute pancreatitis
d. Hypoparathyroidism
e. Thiazide diuretics

3.57 Hypocalcaemia is associated with:

a. Prolongation of the QT interval
b. Acute pancreatitis
c. Paget's disease
d. Addison's disease
e. Pseudohypoparathyroidism

3.58 The following are used in the treatment of hypercalcaemia:

a. Normal saline
b. Steroids
c. Calcitonin
d. Disphosphonates
e. Salicylates

3.59 Regarding hyperkalaemia management:

a. 10 ml of 10% calcium chloride is used
b. Nebulized ipratropium bromide is used in treatment
c. Dialysis is indicated for levels > 6.0
d. Sodium bicarbonate causes K^+ to shift into cells
e. 10 ml of 10% calcium gluconate is used

3.60 Regarding glucagonoma:

a. Associated with diabetes
b. Associated with a migratory rash
c. 50% are malignant
d. Causes weight loss
e. The majority are located in the duodenum

3.61 Regarding causes of diabetes:

a. Acromegaly
b. Phaeochromocytoma
c. Haemochromatosis
d. Peripheral vascular disease
e. Sickle cell disease

3.62 Regarding hyperaldosteronism:

a. Causes a diastolic hypertension
b. Causes a metabolic acidosis
c. Causes hyperkalaemia
d. Causes include renal artery stenosis
e. Adrenal adenoma is the most common cause of primary hyperaldosteronism

3.63 Regarding diabetic ketoacidosis:

a. Serum osmolatity > 320 mosm/kg is associated with a poor prognosis
b. Cerebral oedema is associated with a good long-term prognosis
c. pH < 7.3 and urinary ketones are consistent with the diagnosis
d. All patients require a full septic screen
e. Complications include hypophosphataemia

3.64 Regarding hyperosmolar non-ketotic acidosis:

a. It is associated with a plasma osmolarity > 350 mosm/kg
b. Plasma osmolarity correlates with the degree of reduced consciousness
c. Has a higher mortality rate than diabetic ketoacidosis
d. Typically has a fluid deficit of 8–12 L
e. Associated with an increased risk of thrombosis

3.65 Causes of respiratory alkalosis:

a. Progesterone
b. Nicotine
c. Pneumonia
d. Hyperthyroidism
e. Severe asthma

3.66 Causes of metabolic alkalosis:

a. Massive blood transfusion
b. Cushing's disease
c. Primary and secondary hyperaldosteronism
d. Metformin overdose
e. Diuretics

3.67 Cushing's syndrome associations:

a. Hyperkalaemia
b. Small cell lung cancer
c. Anaplastic thyroid cancer
d. Cataracts
e. Difficulty lifting heavy objects

3.68 Causes of thyrotoxicosis:

a. Iodine
b. Amiodarone
c. Lithium
d. Phenytoin
e. Phenothiazines

3.69 Drugs used in the treatment of thyrotoxic storm:

a. Salicylates
b. Beta-blockers
c. Propylthiouracil
d. Steroids
e. Iodine before propylthiouracil

3.70 Regarding phaeochromocytoma:

a. It requires immediate surgery
b. Beta-blockade should be given before alpha-blockade
c. Can cause a lactic acidosis
d. Crisis may be precipitated by metoclopramide
e. Alpha-blockade should be given before volume rehydration

3.71 Regarding phaeochromocytoma:

a. Derived from chromaffin cells
b. Can cause cardiac arrhythmias
c. Causes hyperkalaemia
d. Associated with hyperparathyroidism
e. Associated with MEN type 1 syndrome

3.72 Cushing's syndrome associations:

a. Metabolic alkalosis
b. Oedema
c. Hyperglycaemia
d. Phaeochromocytoma
e. Hypotension

3.73 Causes of hypercalcaemia:

a. Hypothyroidism
b. AIDS
c. Paget's disease
d. Thiazide diuretics
e. Addison's disease

3.74 Subclavian thrombosis:

a. Is associated with a prominent internal jugular vein
b. Requires anticoagulation
c. Central venous line placement predisposes to this
d. Is associated with non-pitting oedema of the affected limb
e. Is more common in females

3.75 Regarding deep vein thrombosis:

  a. Ileo–femoral thrombus is usually treated on an outpatient basis
  b. High-dose progesterone is a recognized risk factor
  c. Antiphospholipid syndrome predisposes
  d. Aspirin should be given to all patients with a CVA
  e. All patients undergoing long haul air travel should have single dose aspirin pre-travel

3.76 Chronic renal failure is associated with:

  a. Hyperparathyroidism
  b. Hypokalaemia
  c. Impaired platelet function
  d. Pseudo gout
  e. Hypocalcaemia

3.77 Rhabdomyolysis is associated with:

  a. Hyperkalaemia
  b. Raised urate levels
  c. Respiratory acidosis
  d. Treatment includes IV calcium replacement
  e. Treatment includes IV $NaHCO_3$

3.78 Regarding rhabdomyolysis:

  a. Carbon monoxide poisoning is associated
  b. Furosemide is used in management
  c. Mannitol diuresis is used in management
  d. Full recovery of renal function is unlikely
  e. RBC are seen on urine microscopy

3.79 Regarding status epilepticus:

  a. Diazepam has a longer duration of action than lorazepam
  b. Paraldehyde corrodes plastic
  c. Hyponatraemia should be promptly reversed
  d. Glucose replacement should be given before thiamine in alcoholic patients
  e. ECG monitoring should be conducted during phenytoin infusion

3.80 Regarding pseudoseizures:

  a. They are associated with hypoxia
  b. They are associated with hyperprolactinaemia
  c. They are associated with acidosis
  d. Commonly fail to respond to conventional seizure management
  e. Hypoglycaemia can cause these

3.81 Regarding seizures:

a. Associated with hyponatraemia
b. Associated with hypocalcaemia
c. Associated with acute renal failure
d. Associated with amphetamine use
e. Associated with skull fracture

3.82 Regarding hepatic failure:

a. Causes a respiratory acidosis
b. Causes a metabolic alkalosis
c. Splenomegaly is a feature of acute liver failure
d. Causes a macrocytosis
e. Is associated with subconjunctival haemorrhage

3.83 Regarding haematology:

a. Spherocytosis is an autosomal recessive condition
b. Iron absorption increases in the presence of gastric acid
c. Iron is absorbed in the terminal ileum
d. Hypothyroidism causes a macrocytosis
e. Epstein–Barr virus causes aplastic crises in patients with hereditary spherocytosis

3.84 Precipitants of porphyria include:

a. Oestrogens
b. Bupivacaine
c. Barbiturates
d. Ibuprofen
e. Ciprofloxacin

3.85 Regarding porphyria:

a. Is an hereditary condition
b. Causes hyponatraemia
c. Is diagnosed by serum level measurement
d. Causes a motor peripheral neuropathy
e. Can cause psychosis and hallucinations

3.86 Regarding blood groups:

a. Group O is the universal donor
b. Group O is the universal recipient
c. Group A is the most common blood group in the UK
d. A$^+$ blood may be given to an AB$^-$ recipient
e. Full blood compatibility testing takes over 2 hours

3.87 Regarding DIC:

   a. Gram-negative sepsis is a common cause
   b. Associated with increased fibrinogen levels and increased prothrombin time
   c. Can be caused by burns
   d. Associated with thrombocytopenia
   e. Cryoprecipitate is used if fibrinogen levels fall below 200 g/L

3.88 Causes of coma:

   a. Meningism is pathognomonic of meningitis
   b. Arrhythmias may cause coma
   c. Metabolic coma is associated with reactive pupils
   d. Subhyaloid haemorrhage indicates diabetic encephalopathy
   e. Metabolic coma is associated with focal neurological symptoms

3.89 Regarding brainstem death:

   a. Clinical testing should include a member of the transplant team
   b. Tests include assessing the vestibulo-ocular reflex
   c. Tests include assessing the corneal reflex
   d. By definition requires the presence of apnoea
   e. There should be a minimum of 12 hours between tests

3.90 Regarding acute dystonic reactions:

   a. They are a recognized side-effect of metoclopramide
   b. They are a recognized side-effect of risperidone
   c. Procyclidine is used in management
   d. Benztropine is used in management
   e. Atropine is used in management

3.91 Regarding rashes:

   a. Erythema migrans is associated with *Mycoplasma pneumoniae*
   b. Erythema multiforme is associated with *Mycoplasma pneumoniae*
   c. Toxic shock syndrome is associated with a desquamating rash
   d. Kawasaki disease is associated with a desquamating rash
   e. Erythema marginatum is associated with ulcerative colitis

3.92 Regarding Horner's syndrome:

   a. Associated with a dilated pupil
   b. Associated with brachial plexus injuries
   c. Associated with anhydrosis
   d. Associated with enophthamlos
   e. Associated with complete ptosis

3.93 Regarding acute gastroenteritis:

a. Campylobacter infection is treated with erythromycin
b. Re-feeding should commence 24 hours after the last episode
c. Patients with ileostomies have increased risk of dehydration
d. Usually requires intravenous rehydration
e. Oral rehydration therapy is contraindicated in those younger than 3 year olds

3.94 Regarding duodenal ulceration:

a. More common than gastric ulceration
b. Associated with pain on an empty stomach
c. Usually has a recurrent history
d. Ulcers are most commonly located on the posterior duodenal wall
e. Affects 10% of the population

3.95 Characteristics of venous ulcers:

a. Typically lie on the medial aspect of the lower leg
b. Associated with a swollen leg
c. Associated with dry skin
d. Comprise 10% of all ulcers
e. Pain increases with leg elevation

3.96 Common causes of clubbing include:

a. Large cell lung carcinoma
b. Tricuspid atresia
c. Crohn's disease
d. Biliary cirrhosis
e. Hyperparathyroidism

3.97 Causes of gynaecomastia:

a. Cimetidine
b. Spironolactone
c. Phaeochromocytoma
d. Thyrotoxicosis
e. Starvation

3.98 Wernicke's encephalopathy associations:

a. Nystagmus
b. IX cranial nerve palsy
c. Gynaecomastia
d. Papilloedema
e. Neck stiffness

3.99 Causes of hypoglycaemia:

a. Myxoedema
b. Salicylates
c. Beta-blockers

   d. Chlorpromazine
   e. Hyperpituitarism

3.100 Causes of jaundice:

   a. Co-amoxiclav
   b. Phenytoin
   c. Flucloxacillin
   d. Anabolic steroids
   e. Chlorpromazine

3.101 Causes of bloody diarrhoea:

   a. Shigella
   b. Salmonella
   c. *Clostridium difficile*
   d. *E. coli*
   e. Campylobacter

3.1 Answers

a. **True**
b. **True**
c. **False** – plateau pulse is associated with aortic stenosis; aortic regurgitation is associated with a collapsing pulse
d. **True**
e. **True**

3.2 Answers

a. **True**
b. **True**
c. **True**
d. **False** – a third heart sound is often normal during pregnancy or in people younger than 40 years old
e. **True**

3.3 Answers

a. **True**
b. **True**
c. **False** – hypercalcaemia shortens the QT interval
d. **True**
e. **True**

3.4 Regarding sympathetic nerve supply:

a. **True**
b. **False** – sympathetic nerve supply causes pupillary dilatation
c. **True**
d. **True**
e. **True**

3.5 Answers

a. **True**
b. **False** – small cell lung carcinoma is usually not associated with clubbing
c. **True**
d. **True**
e. **False**

3.6 Answers

a. **True** – if pulmonary hypertension is also present
b. **True** – if atrial fibrillation is also present
c. **True**
d. **True**
e. **False** – mitral stenosis is associated with a diastolic murmur

3.7 Answers

a. **True**
b. **True**
c. **True**
d. **False**
e. **False**

3.8 Answers

a. **True** – Hill's sign is higher blood pressure in the legs compared to the arms
b. **False**
c. **True**
d. **True** – Quincke's sign is the visible pulsation seen in the finger nail bed
e. **False** – Phalen's sign is a sign of carpal tunnel syndrome

3.9 Answers

a. **True**
b. **True**
c. **True**
d. **True** – often associated with aortic regurgitation
e. **True**

3.10 Answers

a. **True**
b. **True**
c. **True**
d. **False** – complete heart block causes cannon A waves
e. **False** – tricuspid regurgitation causes enlarged V waves

3.11 Answers

a. **False**
b. **True**
c. **True**
d. **False**
e. **False**

3.12 Answers

a. **True**
b. **True** – hydralazine increases risk of pericarditis
c. **False**
d. **False** – concave upward ST segments
e. **True**

3.13 Answers

a. **True**
b. **True**
c. **False** – subendocardial myocardial infarction is associated with ST depression and deeply inverted T waves
d. **False** – right ventricular failure usually requires fluids to achieve adequate filling pressures
e. **True**

3.14 Answers

a. **True**
b. **False** – digoxin shortens the QT interval
c. **True**
d. **False** – hypothermia can prolong the QT interval
e. **True** – imipramine is a tricyclic antidepressant

3.15 Answers

a. **True**
b. **False** – atrial filling with a closed tricuspid valve describes the V wave; the C wave occurs when the tricuspid valve enters the atrium during ventricular contraction
c. **False** – atrial fibrillation is associated with absent A waves
d. **True**
e. **True**

3.16 Answers

a. **True** – due to risk of hypotension
b. **True**
c. **False**
d. **False** – aim for a 30% blood pressure drop
e. **False** – sodium nitroprusside is light sensitive

3.17 Answers

a. **True**
b. **True**
c. **False** – left ventricular ejection fraction <40 % is an indication for ACE inhibitor use
d. **True** – ACE inhibitors may cause fetal injury or death
e. **False** – reduced doses of ACE inhibitors are required in renal failure; avoid in bilateral renal artery stenosis

3.18 Answers

a. **True**
b. **True**
c. **False**
d. **False** – beta-blockers are contraindicated if SBP < 100 mmHg
e. **True**

3.19 Answers

a. **True**
b. **True**
c. **False**
d. **True**
e. **False**

3.20 Answers

a. **True**
b. **False**
c. **True** – useful for arrhythmias known to be of supraventricular origin
d. **False** – calcium channel blockers should be avoided in atrial fibrillation and WPW
e. **True**

3.21 Answers

a. **False** – calcium channel blockers are contraindicated in WPW
b. **False** – U waves are associated with hypokalaemia; delta waves are associated with WPW
c. **True**
d. **True**
e. **True** – and an inverted T wave in the anterior leads

3.22 Answers

a. **True**
b. **True**
c. **True**
d. **True**
e. **True**

3.23 Answers

a. **True**
b. **True** – carotid sinus pressure causes an uncoupling of the atria and ventricles, often revealing flutter waves
c. **True**
d. **True** – the atria often beat at a rate of exactly 300 bpm; when associated with 2:1 block a rate of 150 bpm is seen. Atrial flutter should always be considered in a narrow complex tachycardia with a rate of 150 bpm
e. **False** – sotalol is used in the management of atrial flutter although all antiarrhythmics carry a risk of inducing an arrhythmias

3.24 Answers

a. **False** – sotalol may lengthen the QT interval causing torsades de pointes
b. **True**
c. **False**
d. **False** – fusion beats are associated with ventricular tachycardia
e. **False**

3.25 Answers

a. **True**
b. **True**
c. **True**
d. **True**
e. **False**

3.26 Answers

a. **True**
b. **True**
c. **True**
d. **True**
e. **True**

3.27 Answers

a. **True**
b. **True** – pulselessness is associated with ventricular fibrillation
c. **True**
d. **True**
e. **False** – heart rate > 150 bpm

3.28 Answers

a. **False** – adenosine would exacerbate the bradycardia; atropine is used
b. **True**
c. **True**
d. **True**
e. **True**

3.29 Answers

a. **False** – Mg^{2+} should be given as first line unless the patient is haemodynamically compromised
b. **False** – verapamil may cause hypotension
c. **True**
d. **True**
e. **True**

3.30 Answers

a. **True**
b. **True**
c. **False** – IV opioids are useful; they reduce preload
d. **True**
e. **False** – hypotensive patients require inotropic support, e.g. with dobutamine; aggressive fluid resuscitation may aggravate the problem

3.31 Answers

a. **True**
b. **True** – secondary to neurotoxicity from medications or from immune-mediated glomerulonephritis
c. **True**
d. **False** – if the source of infection is *Staph. aureus* there is a high risk of intracerebral haemorrhage rendering anticoagulation dangerous
e. **True**

3.32 Answers

a. **True**
b. **False**
c. **True** – if uraemia causes cardiac tamponade
d. **False**
e. **True**

3.33 Answers

a. **False** – the pulmonary congestion may be due to reduced ventricular compliance from ischaemia
b. **False**
c. **True**
d. **True**
e. **True** – unless calcium antagonists are used in conjunction with beta-blockers or nitrates

3.34 Answers

a. **True**
b. **True**
c. **True**
d. **True**
e. **True**

3.35 Answers

a. **False** – A–V block is a contraindication for beta-blockade
b. **True**
c. **False**
d. **True**
e. **False**

3.36 Answers

a. **True**
b. **True**
c. **False** – ulcerative colitis and acute myocardial infarction is a relative contraindication
d. **False** – renal disease and acute myocardial infarction is a contraindication
e. **True** – This indicates impaired left ventricular function

3.37 Answers

a. **True**
b. **True**
c. **True**
d. **True**
e. **True** – usually the posterior papillary muscle and typically at day 2–10

3.38 Answers

a. **True**
b. **True**
c. **True**
d. **False** – episodes of bradycardia should only be treated if associated with hypotension or a rate of < 50 bpm
e. **True**

3.39 Answers

a. **True**
b. **False** – central rather than peripheral cyanosis is usually seen in severe asthma
c. **True**
d. **True**
e. **False** – PEF of 50% of predicted value often occurs in severe asthma

3.40 Answers

a. **False** – only low- and intermediate-risk patients should have D-dimer test
b. **False**
c. **True**
d. **True**
e. **True**

3.41 Answers

a. **False** – immediate treatment risks worsening the clinical condition
b. **False** – a CXR should be performed only if pneumothorax or consolidation is suspected
c. **True**
d. **True**
e. **False** – IV aminophylline is used in the management of acute severe asthma

3.42 Answers

a. **True**
b. **False** – $PaCO_2$ <4.6 kPA is expected for life-threatening asthma
c. **True**
d. **False** – inability to complete full sentences is a sign of acute severe asthma
e. **False** – PEF 33–50% is a sign of acute severe asthma; in life-threatening asthma a PEF of < 33% of best or predicted would be expected

3.43 Answers

a. **True**
b. **True**
c. **False**
d. **False** – excessive coughing is a sign of failed aspiration
e. **True**

3.44 Answers

a. **True**
b. **False** – secondary pneumothorax tends to have more severe symptoms than primary pneumothorax
c. **True** – it increases the rate of resorption x 4
d. **False** – diving is contraindicated unless bilateral surgical pleurectomy has been performed
e. **False** – patients should be observed overnight

3.45 Answers

a. **True**
b. **False** – *Strep. pneumoniae* is the most common bacterial cause of pneumonia
c. **False** – PaO_2 of < 8 kPa is a poor prognostic indicator
d. **True** – urea > 7 is a poor prognostic indicator
e. **True**

3.46 Answers

a. **True** – the pH is low, the $PaCO_2$ is raised, and the HCO_3 is normal
b. **False**
c. **False** – this ABG would cause a metabolic alkalosis
d. **True**

3.47 Answers

a. **True** – the pH is raised, the $PaCO_2$ is normal, and the HCO_3 is raised
b. **True**
c. **False**
d. **True**

3.48 Answers

a. **True** – this ABG shows a fully compensated respiratory acidosis; the pH is low normal, the HCO_3 is raised, and the $PaCO_2$ is raised
b. **True**
c. **False**
d. **True**

3.49 Answers

a. **True** – this ABG shows a partially compensated metabolic acidosis; the pH, $PaCO_2$, and HCO_3 are all low
b. **False**
c. **False**
d. **False**

3.50 Answers

a. **False** – this shows a fully compensated metabolic alkalosis
b. **True**
c. **False** – this shows a fully compensated respiratory acidosis; the HCO_3 is returning to baseline values
d. **False** – this shows a metabolic alkalosis

3.51 Answers

a. **True**
b. **True**
c. **True**
d. **True**
e. **False**

3.52 Answers

a. **True**
b. **False** – pyloric stenosis causes hypokalaemia
c. **True**
d. **True**
e. **False** – excess liquorice intake causes hypokalaemia

3.53 Answers

    a. True – associated with levels > 7.0
    b. True – associated with levels > 8.0
    c. True
    d. False – delta waves are seen in patients with WPW syndrome
    e. False – U waves are seen in hypokalaemia

3.54 Answers

    a. True
    b. True
    c. True
    d. True
    e. True

3.55 Answers

    a. True
    b. True
    c. True
    d. False – diabetes insipidus causes hypernatraemia
    e. False – primary hyperaldosteronism causes hypernatraemia

3.56 Answers

    a. False – tetany is associated with hypocalcaemia
    b. False – Trousseau's sign is associated with hypocalcaemia
    c. False – acute pancreatitis is associated with hypocalcaemia
    d. False – hypoparathyroidism is associated with hypocalcaemia
    e. True

3.57 Answers

    a. True
    b. True
    c. False – Paget's disease is associated with hypercalcaemia
    d. False – Addison's disease is associated with hypercalcaemia
    e. True

3.58 Answers

    a. True
    b. True
    c. True
    d. True
    e. False

3.59 Answers

    a. True
    b. False – nebulized salbutamol is used
    c. False – dialysis is indicated for levels > 7.0
    d. True
    e. True

3.60 Answers

a. **True**
b. **True**
c. **True**
d. **True**
e. **False** – this is a tumour of the alpha 2 cells of the islets of Langerhans

3.61 Answers

a. **True**
b. **True**
c. **True**
d. **False** – diabetes causes peripheral vascular disease
e. **False**

3.62 Answers

a. **True**
b. **False** – hyperaldosteronism causes a metabolic alkalosis
c. **False** – hyperaldosteronism causes hypokalaemia
d. **True**
e. **True** – in up to 60% of cases

3.63 Answers

a. **True**
b. **False** – up to 70% of patients with cerebral oedema die
c. **True**
d. **True** – 30% of cases are secondary to infection
e. **True** – phosphate enters cells with K^+

3.64 Answers

a. **True**
b. **True**
c. **True**
d. **True**
e. **True**

3.65 Answers

a. **True** – due to stimulation of the respiratory centre
b. **True**
c. **True** – stimulates the chest receptors
d. **True**
e. **False** – severe asthma causes respiratory acidosis

3.66 Answers

a. **True** – due to citrate metabolism
b. **True**
c. **True**
d. **False** – metformin overdose causes a lactic acidosis
e. **True** – diuretics cause the loss of H^+ in the kidneys by increasing the H^+–K^+ exchange in the distal convoluted tubule

3.67 Answers

a. **False** – Cushing's syndrome is associated with hypokalaemia
b. **True** – through ectopic ACTH secretion
c. **False** – Cushing's syndrome is associated with medullary thyroid cancer
d. **True**
e. **True** – due to proximal myopathy

3.68 Answers

a. **True**
b. **True**
c. **True**
d. **False** – phenytoin may interact with thyroxine and increase thyroxine degradation
e. **False**

3.69 Answers

a. **False** – salicylates are contraindicated as they can displace T4
b. **True**
c. **True**
d. **True**
e. **False** – propylthiouracil should be used first to block the organification of iodine; otherwise iodine may increase thyroid hormone stores

3.70 Answers

a. **False** – surgery is dangerous before adequate rehydration and appropriate alpha- and beta-blockade
b. **False** – alpha-blockade should be administered before beta-blockade
c. **True**
d. **True**
e. **False** – alpha-blockade given first would risk hypotension

3.71 Answers

a. **True**
b. **True**
c. **False** – phaeochromocytoma causes hypokalaemia
d. **True**
e. **False** – phaeochromocytoma is associated with MEN type 2 syndrome

3.72 Answers

a. **True**
b. **True**
c. **True**
d. **True**
e. **False** – Cushing's syndrome is associated with hypertension

3.73 Answers

a. **False**
b. **True**
c. **True**
d. **True**
e. **True**

3.74 Answers

a. **False** – a prominent internal jugular vein would indicate superior vena cava obstruction
b. **True** – to prevent progression of the clot
c. **True**
d. **True**
e. **False**

3.75 Answers

a. **False** – ileo-femoral thrombus is usually treated as an inpatient due to high risk of pulmonary embolus
b. **True**
c. **True**
d. **False** – some patients with a haemorrhagic CVA are excluded from aspirin
e. **False** – only high-risk patients should take aspirin pre-travel

3.76 Answers

a. **True**
b. **False** – hyperkalaemia is associated with chronic renal failure
c. **True**
d. **True**
e. **True**

3.77 Answers

a. **True**
b. **True**
c. **False** – metabolic acidosis is associated with rhabdomyolysis
d. **False** – IV calcium replacement can cause metastatic calcium deposition in damaged muscle and tissue necrosis
e. **True** – IV $NaHCO_3$ causes urinary alkalinization which increases the solubility of myoglobin

3.78 Answers

a. **True**
b. **False** – furosemide may acidify the urine and increase myoglobin-induced tubular damage
c. **True**
d. **False** – full recovery of renal function is likely
e. **False** – myoglobin in urine causes a false-positive result on dipstick

3.79 Answers

a. **False** – lorazepam has a longer duration of action than diazepam
b. **True**
c. **False** – hyponatraemia should be reversed cautiously due to the risk of precipitating pontine myelinosis
d. **False** – thiamine should be administered first as glucose increases the risk of Wernicke's encephalopathy
e. **True** – due to the risk of arrhythmias

3.80 Answers

a. **False** – hypoxia indicates genuine seizures
b. **False** – hyperprolactinaemia indicates genuine seizures
c. **False** – acidosis indicates genuine seizures
d. **True**
e. **False** – hypoglycaemia would cause a genuine seizure

3.81 Answers

a. **True**
b. **True**
c. **True** – seizures are associated with uraemia
d. **True**
e. **True**

3.82 Answers

a. **True**
b. **True**
c. **False** – splenomegaly is a sign of chronic liver failure
d. **True**
e. **True** – highest incidence of subconjunctival haemorrhage in paracetamol induced liver failure

3.83 Answers

a. **False** – spherocytosis is an autosomal dominant condition
b. **True**
c. **False** – vitamin B_{12} is absorbed in the terminal ileum; iron is absorbed in the duodenum and jejunum
d. **True**
e. **False** – parvovirus causes aplastic crises in patients with hereditary spherocytosis

3.84 Answers

a. **True**
b. **False**
c. **True**
d. **False**
e. **False**

3.85 Answers

a. **True** – can also be acquired in lead poisoning, iron deficiency and alcohol excess
b. **True**
c. **False** – diagnosis is made by urinalysis measuring porphobilinogen concentration
d. **True**
e. **True**

3.86 Answers

a. **True**
b. **False** – group AB⁺ is the universal recipient
c. **False** – O 46%; A 42%; AB 3%; B 9%
d. **False**
e. **False** – may take up to 1 hour

3.87 Answers

a. **True** – 60% of cases are caused by sepsis
b. **False** – prothrombin time increases but fibrinogen levels fall via thrombin activation
c. **True**
d. **True**
e. **True**

3.88 Answers

a. **False** – meningism is also seen in patients with subarachnoid haemorrhage and encephalitis
b. **True** – if the arrhythmias cause poor cerebral perfusion
c. **True** – unless secondary to atropine overdose which depresses the brainstem function and causes pupillary abnormalities
d. **False** – subhyaloid haemorrhages are seen with subarachnoid haemorrhage
e. **False** – focal neurological symptoms are rarely seen in patients with metabolic coma; this is more typical of structural lesions

3.89 Answers

a. **False** – the transplant team should not be involved in the assessment for the presence of brainstem death
b. **True**
c. **True**
d. **True**
e. **False** – there is no minimum time lag between testing

3.90 Answers

a. **True**
b. **True**
c. **True**
d. **True**
e. **False**

3.91 Answers

a. **False** – erythema migrans is associated with Lyme's disease
b. **True**
c. **True**
d. **True**
e. **False** – erythema marginatum is associated with rheumatic fever

3.92 Answers

a. **False** – Horner's syndrome is associated with miosis due to paralysis of the sympathetically innervated Muller's muscle which usually dilates the pupil
b. **True** – if the T1 nerve root is involved
c. **True** – the absence of sweating
d. **False**
e. **False** – Horner's syndrome is associated with partial ptosis

3.93 Answers

a. **True** – if there is associated systemic upset
b. **False** – re-feeding should commence as soon as possible after the last episode of acute gastroenteritis
c. **True**
d. **False** – oral rehydration is adequate for the majority of patients with acute gastroenteritis
e. **False**

3.94 Answers

a. **True**
b. **True**
c. **True**
d. **True**
e. **True**

3.95 Answers

a. **True**
b. **True**
c. **True**
d. **False** – 70% of all ulcers are venous ulcers; 10% are ischaemic in origin
e. **False** – increased pain with leg elevation is characteristic of ischaemic ulcers

3.96 Answers

a. **True**
b. **False** – tricuspid atresia is not a common cause although it may cause clubbing
c. **True**
d. **True**
e. **False**

3.97 Answers

a. **True**
b. **True**
c. **False**
d. **True**
e. **True** – due to increased oestrogen production in starvation

3.98 Answers

a. **True**
b. **False** – Wernicke's encephalopathy is associated with cranial nerve VI palsy
c. **True**
d. **False** – papilloedema is a sign of raised intracranial pressure
e. **False** – neck stiffness is a sign of meningism

3.99 Answers

a. **True**
b. **True**
c. **True**
d. **False**
e. **False** – hyperpituitarism is associated with diabetes

3.100 Answers

a. **True**
b. **True**
c. **True**
d. **True**
e. **True**

3.101 Answers

a. **True**
b. **True**
c. **True**
d. **True** – enterotoxogenic *E. coli*
e. **True**

4. Toxicology

4.1 Toxicology syndromes:

a. Paraquat-induced hypoxia requires oxygen
b. Hyper-reflexia, tachycardia and dilated pupils are associated with TCA overdose
c. Extensor plantar response is associated with paraquat overdose
d. Tachycardia, hyperventilation and tinnitus are associated with paracetamol overdose
e. Tinnitus, divergent squint and coma are associated with TCA overdose

4.2 Toxicology associations:

a. Salicylate overdose and hyperthermia
b. TCA and cocaine overdose are associated with seizures
c. Anticholinergic overdose is associated with hyperthermia
d. Class 1A and 1C antiarrhythmics cause QRS complex prolongation
e. Ca^{2+} channel blockers are associated with hypotension

4.3 Drug characteristics suitable for haemodialysis:

a. Low molecular weight
b. Large volume of distribution
c. High plasma protein binding
d. High water solubility
e. Unionized drugs

4.4 Activated charcoal:

a. Is used in lithium overdose
b. Is used in digoxin overdose
c. Is used for drugs that are toxic in large quantities
d. Is 'activated' by treatment in acid or steam at high temperatures
e. Is contraindicated in the presence of an unprotected airway

4.5 Haemoperfusion complications:

a. Hypotension
b. Hypocalcaemia
c. Thrombocytopenia
d. Air embolus
e. Hypercalcaemia

4.6   Indications for gastric lavage:

a. Alkalotic drugs
b. Anticholinergic drugs
c. Ingestions more than 6 hours old
d. Patients with unprotected airways
e. Patients with a low Glasgow Coma Scale

4.7   Regarding drug overdoses:

a. Physostigmine is a short-acting acetylcholinesterase inhibitor
b. Conduction delay is a contraindication to physostigmine
c. Anticholinergic overdose is associated with mydriasis
d. Occurrence of seizures after anticholinergic overdose is a poor prognostic indicator
e. Serum levels are useful in anticholinergic overdose

4.8   The following drug and antidotes are associated:

a. Glucagon and beta-blockers
b. $NaHCO_3$ and atropine
c. Flumazenil and opioids
d. Diazepam and chloroquine
e. Iron and desferoxamine

4.9   The following drug and antidotes are associated:

a. Ethanol and ethylene glycol
b. Methylene blue and methanol
c. Amylnitrate and cyanide
d. Oxygen and carbon monoxide
e. Insulin and sulphonylurea

4.10   Regarding iron overdose:

a. May be diagnosed by abdominal ultrasound
b. Plain abdominal X-rays help with diagnosis
c. Absence of tablets on plain X-ray rules out overdose
d. IV nitroprusside is used to manage hypertension if it occurs
e. Lithium and potassium are radio-opaque

4.11   Regarding digoxin toxicity:

a. Is associated with hypokalaemia
b. Serum levels of >15 mmol/L are an indication for the use of digoxin-specific FAb antibodies
c. Causes reduced vagal tone
d. Is renally excreted
e. Ingestion of > 10 mg is an indication for digoxin-specific FAb antibodies

4.12   **Regarding iron overdose:**

   a. It is irritative to the gastric mucosa
   b. Can cause small bowel obstruction
   c. In pregnancy is associated with abortion and preterm labour
   d. Chelation treatment causes iron redistribution into plasma from tissues
   e. Gastrointestinal symptoms occur before systemic toxicity

4.13   **Regarding methanol overdose:**

   a. Ethanol is used in treatment
   b. It can cause blindness
   c. Aim of treatment is to stop the metabolism of methanol
   d. Causes photophobia
   e. Folic acid is used in management

4.14   **Regarding paracetamol overdose:**

   a. N-acetylcysteine (NAC) is hepatically metabolized to cysteine
   b. Malnourished patients have increased risk of toxicity
   c. Patients on carbamazepine have increased risk of toxicity
   d. IV methionine may be used in treatment instead of NAC
   e. NAC acts as a substrate for hepatic sulphation

4.15   **Regarding paracetamol overdose:**

   a. Jaundice appears during the first 24 hours of overdose
   b. Levels of > 200 mg/L at 4 hours have a 60% chance of hepatotoxicity without treatment
   c. Patients presenting at 9 hours post overdose, having taken > 150 mg/L should have NAC
   d. Patients with deteriorating liver function tests at 20 hours should have ongoing NAC
   e. ALT is the first liver enzyme to increase post overdose

4.16   **Regarding paracetamol overdose:**

   a. Methionine or NAC can be used post activated charcoal ingestion
   b. Paracetamol is predominately renally metabolized
   c. 60% of paracetamol is conjugated to glutathione
   d. Overdose causes a centrilobular hepatic necrosis
   e. A rising prothrombin time at day 4 indicates increased risk of fulminant hepatic failure

4.17   **Regarding lithium overdose:**

   a. Levels correlate with degree of clinical severity
   b. Toxicity is associated with hyper-reflexia and ataxia
   c. Dehydration predisposes to toxicity
   d. Symptoms usually occur within 12 hours of overdose
   e. ACE inhibitors predispose to toxicity

4.18   Regarding salicylate overdose:

    a. Overdose causes hyperventilation
    b. Causes a metabolic alkalosis initially
    c. Levels > 300 mg/kg are fatal
    d. Levels < 200 mg/kg are safe and allow the patient to be safely discharged
    e. Renal excretion is maximum with an acidic urine pH

4.19   Regarding salicylate overdose:

    a. Associated with dehydration and hyperpyrexia
    b. Hypokalaemia is an indication for haemodialysis
    c. Treatment should aim for a urine pH > 7.5
    d. Normokalaemia is desirable in treatment
    e. Persistent acidosis is an indication for haemodialysis

4.20   Tricyclic antidepressants:

    a. Cause sodium channel blockade
    b. Are associated with ventricular tachyarrhythmias
    c. Levels correlate accurately with the severity of poisoning
    d. Degree of QRS prolongation correlates with the risk of ventricular arrhythmias
    e. Cause hypotension due to their alpha-adrenergic effects

4.21   Regarding amphetamines:

    a. Associated with intracerebral haemorrhage
    b. Causes hypernatraemia
    c. Associated with hypothermia
    d. Act as sympathomimetics
    e. Use can lead to tolerance

4.22   Tricyclic antidepressants:

    a. A QRS duration of 120 ms is considered cardiotoxic
    b. $NaHCO_3$ is used in the management of overdose
    c. Dialysis is effective in the management of overdose
    d. Flumazenil is recommended in the management of overdose
    e. Pralidoxime is effective in the management of overdose

4.23   Cocaine:

    a. Is a sympathomimetic
    b. Is a vasodilator
    c. Shortens the QT interval
    d. Is associated with pneumothorax
    e. Has been used as a local anaesthetic in the past

4.24 Regarding cyanide poisoning:

a. Causes a lactic acidosis
b. Causes a ketoacidosis
c. Associated with excessive sodium nitroprusside use
d. Treatment options includes dicobalt edetate
e. Hydroxocobalamin treatment complexes with cyanide to form cynacobalamin

4.25 Regarding cocaine:

a. Associated with increased risk of cerebrovascular attack
b. Associated with increased risk of coronary artery disease
c. Associated with photophobia
d. Is detectable on urinalysis for 1 week after use
e. Associated with significant risk of myocardial infarction in the first hour after use

4.26 Regarding organophosphate overdose:

a. Treatments include IV atropine
b. Treatments include IV adenosine
c. Are associated with respiratory failure
d. Organophosphates may be absorbed through skin and bronchi
e. Causes acetylcholinesterase accumulation

4.27 Regarding methaemoglobinaemia:

a. Nitrates predispose to this
b. Sulphonamides predispose to this
c. Can be an inherited or an acquired condition
d. Methylene blue is a known causative agent
e. Causes a cyanosis unresponsive to oxygen therapy

4.28 Regarding methaemoglobinaemia:

a. Diagnosis is made by spectrophotometry
b. Methylene blue is used in management
c. If the correct diagnosis is made methylene blue is always effective in management
d. Causes a right shift of the oxygen–haemoglobin dissociation curve
e. Oxygen saturations are a reliable indicator of the degree of hypoxia

4.29 Regarding hypoglycaemic drug overdose:

a. Octreotide is used in metformin overdose
b. Octreotide blocks insulin release from beta cells
c. Sulphonylurea overdose causes lactic acidosis
d. Chronic renal failure predisposes to lactic acidosis in metformin overdose
e. Sulphonylureas are hepatically metabolized

4.30 Regarding beta-blocker overdose:

a. Causes syncope
b. Treatment includes use of an antimuscarinic agent
c. Causes hypertension
d. Can cause heart failure
e. Treatment may involve use of adenosine

4.31 Regarding CO poisoning:

a. CO is produced by incomplete combustion of hydrocarbons
b. Causes rightward shift of the oxygen–haemoglobin dissociation curve
c. Poisoning is more severe if the patient is anaemic
d. Causes ST depression on ECG
e. Binds haemoglobin with 40 times more affinity than oxygen

4.32 Regarding CO poisoning:

a. CO binds myoglobin
b. Levels of > 50% are fatal
c. All patients should receive hyperbaric treatment
d. Arterial blood gases are diagnostic
e. Hyperbaric treatment has a risk of barotrauma

4.1 Answers

a. **False** – oxygen increases the toxicity of paraquat
b. **True**
c. **False** – extensor plantar response is associated with TCA overdose
d. **False** – tachycardia, hyperventilation, and tinnitus are associated with aspirin overdose
e. **False** – TCA overdose does not cause tinnitus

4.2 Answers

a. **True**
b. **True**
c. **True** – and also with hypertension
d. **True**
e. **True**

4.3 Answers

a. **True**
b. **False**
c. **False**
d. **True**
e. **True** – e.g. lithium

4.4 Answers

a. **False** – lithium does not bind to activated charcoal
b. **True**
c. **False** – a 10:1 ratio is needed to absorb all toxins; it is ideal for drugs that are toxic in small quantities, e.g. digoxin
d. **True**
e. **True**

4.5 Answers

a. **True**
b. **True**
c. **True**
d. **True**
e. **False**

4.6 Answers

a. **False** – alkalotic drugs are a contraindication to gastric lavage
b. **True** – anticholinergic drugs decrease gastric mobility
c. **False** – gastric lavage works best on recent ingestions
d. **False** – an unprotected airway is a contraindication to gastric lavage
e. **True**

4.7 Answers

a. **True**
b. **True** – due to risk of asystole
c. **True**
d. **True** – central manifestations such as seizures are poor prognostic indicators
e. **False** – no serum level markers are useful in anticholinergic overdose

4.8 Answers

a. **True**
b. **False** – physostigmine is used in atropine overdose
c. **False** – naloxone is used in opioid overdose
d. **True**
e. **True**

4.9 Answers

a. **True**
b. **False** – methylene blue is used in methaemoglobinaemia
c. **True**
d. **True**
e. **False** – dextrose is used in sulphonylurea overdose

4.10 Answers

a. **False**
b. **True**
c. **False** – tablets may have disintegrated
d. **True** – useful as IV nitroprusside is short acting
e. **True**

4.11 Answers

a. **True**
b. **True**
c. **False** – digoxin is associated with increased vagal tone
d. **True**
e. **True**

4.12 Answers

a. **True**
b. **True** – due to gastrointestinal scarring secondary to iron's corrosive effects
c. **True**
d. **True**
e. **True**

4.13 Answers

    a. **True**
    b. **True** – via damage to the optic nerve
    c. **True** – methanol overdose is toxic due to its metabolites
    d. **True**
    e. **True** – used intravenously to prevent optic nerve damage in significant methanol overdoses

4.14 Answers

    a. **True** – cysteine is a precursor to glutathione
    b. **True** – due to glutathione deficiency
    c. **True** – due to enhanced microsomal metabolism
    d. **False** – methionine is given orally not intravenously
    e. **True**

4.15 Answers

    a. **False** – jaundice occurs at 2–4 days post paracetamol overdose
    b. **True**
    c. **True**
    d. **True** – until levels normalize
    e. **False** – prothrombin time rises first; ALT rises at day 3–4

4.16 Answers

    a. **False** – as methionine is given orally it is not recommended
    b. **False** – paracetamol is predominately hepatically metabolized
    c. **False** – paracetamol conjugates to glucuronide metabolites
    d. **True**
    e. **True**

4.17 Answers

    a. **False** – patient's clinical state is often worse than the serum levels suggest
    b. **True**
    c. **True**
    d. **False** – may take 24 hours for symptoms of lithium overdose to be seen, especially with slow-release tablets
    e. **True** – ACE inhibitors reduce renal elimination of lithium due to their effect on renal tubular re-absorption of sodium

4.18 Answers

    a. **True**
    b. **False** – salicylate overdose causes an initial respiratory alkalosis
    c. **False** – levels > 500 mg/kg are considered life threatening
    d. **False** – patients with levels < 150 mg/kg may be safely discharged
    e. **False** – an alkaline urine maximizes urinary excretion

4.19 Answers

a. **True**
b. **False** – hyperkalaemia of > 7.2 mmol/L is an indication for haemodialysis
c. **True**
d. **True**
e. **True**

4.20 Answers

a. **True** – this causes prolongation of the QRS complex
b. **True**
c. **False**
d. **True**
e. **True**

4.21 Answers

a. **True**
b. **False** – hyponatraemia is associated with amphetamines
c. **False** – amphetamines cause hyperthermia
d. **True**
e. **True**

4.22 Answers

a. **True**
b. **True** – to help overcome the sodium channel blockade and hence cardiotoxicity
c. **False** – dialysis is not suitable due to its large volume of distribution
d. **False** – flumazenil may cause refractory seizures
e. **False** – pralidoxime is used in organophosphate overdose

4.23 Answers

a. **True**
b. **False** – cocaine is a vasoconstrictor
c. **False** – cocaine prolongs the QT interval
d. **True** – if smoked
e. **True**

4.24 Answers

a. **True**
b. **False**
c. **True**
d. **True**
e. **True**

4.25 Answers

a. **True** – as it is a potent vasoconstrictor
b. **True** – long-term use is associated with the build-up of atheroma
c. **True** – crack (the smokable form of cocaine) is associated with photophobia
d. **False** – cocaine's metabolites are detectable for 2–3 days post ingestion
e. **True** – one study showed an increased risk of 23 fold in the first hour post use

4.26 Answers

a. **True**
b. **False**
c. **True**
d. **True**
e. **True** – via cholinesterase inhibition

4.27 Answers

a. **True**
b. **True**
c. **True**
d. **True** – if excessive doses are given methylene blue acts as an oxidant and worsens the methylene blue
e. **True**

4.28 Answers

a. **True**
b. **True**
c. **False** – methylene blue is not effective if the patient is deficient of glucose-6-phosphate dehydrogenase; exchange transfusion should be used for these patients
d. **False** – methaemoglobinaemia causes a left shift of the oxygen–haemoglobin dissociation curve
e. **False** – methaemoglobin is absorbed at the same wavelength as oxyhaemoglobin and therefore may have artificially high readings

4.29 Answers

a. **False** – octreotide is used in sulphonylurea overdose
b. **True** – octreotide blocks the action of sulphonylureas
c. **False** – metformin overdose causes lactic acidosis
d. **True** – due to drug accumulation due to decreased renal excretion
e. **True** – metformin is renally metabolized

4.30 Answers

a. **True**
b. **True** – atropine if severe bradycardia is present (< 40 bpm)
c. **False** – beta-blocker overdose causes hypotension
d. **True**
e. **False** – atropine may be used, not adenosine

4.31 Answers

a. **True**
b. **False** – CO poisoning causes a left shift of the oxygen–haemoglobin dissociation curve
c. **True**
d. **True**
e. **False** – CO binds haemoglobin with 240 times greater affinity than oxygen

4.32 Answers

a. **True**
b. **False** – levels of > 70% are fatal
c. **False** – due to the associated risks, such as hyperoxic seizures, not all patients are suitable for hyperbaric treatment
d. **False** – arterial blood gases do not distinguish oxyhaemoglobin from carboxyhaemoglobin; however, they would show an acidosis
e. **True**

5. Paediatrics

5.1 Regarding normal childhood development:

a. 3 months old: able to transfer objects
b. 6 months old: able to turn head to sound
c. 1 year old: has 1–2 words
d. 2 years old: builds tower of seven bricks
e. 21–24 months: joins words to form sentence

5.2 Signs of acute severe asthma in children older than 5 years:

a. SpO_2 < 92%
b. Heart rate > 120 bpm
c. PEF 55% of best or predicted value
d. Silent chest
e. Respiratory rate 12 breaths/min

5.3 Regarding asthma in children:

a. Skin allergy testing often diagnoses the precipitating cause
b. Pulmonary function testing is used in children older than 4 years
c. Steroid inhalers have immediate bronchodilator effect
d. Salbutamol acts on adrenergic receptors
e. FEV_1 shows airway obstruction more reliably than PEF

5.4 Regarding childhood asthma:

a. Inhaled steroids often stunt growth
b. Outdoor exercises should be avoided over the winter months
c. 50% of children outgrow the disease
d. Prevention drug of choice is sodium chromoglycate
e. Persistent cough is often the only symptom

5.5 Regarding bronchiolitis:

a. At-risk groups include frequent attenders at A&E
b. Preterm infants have increased susceptibility
c. Children with associated wheeze should have bronchodilator therapy
d. Children with crackles on auscultation should have a CXR
e. Physiotherapy has been shown to be beneficial in the acute phase

5.6 Regarding Emla cream:

a. Contains lignocaine and bupivacaine
b. Contraindicated in patients younger than 1 year old
c. Contraindicated in patients with haemochromatosis
d. Contraindicated in patients with methaemoglobinaemia
e. Contraindicated in patients with phaeochromocytoma

5.7 Regarding seizures in children:

a. IV lorazepam is contraindicated due to the risk of respiratory depression
b. Buccal midazolam may be used if IV access is not available
c. A pyrexia at presentation indicates a febrile convulsion and no further investigations are warranted
d. Status epilepticus is more common in children than in adults
e. Patients on regular phenytoin should be commenced on a phenytoin infusion if they fail to respond to benzodiazepines

5.8 Regarding seizures in children:

a. IV lorazepam is contraindicated due to the risk of respiratory depression
b. Buccal midazolam may be used if IV access is not available
c. If pyrexial at the time of seizure no further investigations are required
d. Status epilepticus is more common in children than in adults
e. Patients on regular phenytoin should be commenced on a phenytoin infusion if they fail to respond to benzodiazepines

5.9 Regarding hypertrophic pyloric stenosis:

a. Associated with bile-stained vomit
b. Associated with hypochloraemic acidosis
c. Associated with loss of appetite
d. Requires immediate surgical intervention
e. Patients have a palpable abdominal mass during a test feed

5.10 Regarding intussusception:

a. Commonly occurs between 3 and 5 years of age
b. Associated with an abdominal mass
c. Patient may be pain free in between episodes
d. There is an increased incidence in patients with hypertrophic pyloric stenosis
e. Barium enemas are contraindicated; air enemas are used in preference

5.11 Regarding genital problems in childhood:

    a. Foreskin usually remains non-retractile until age 10 years
    b. Balanitis requires treatment with IV antibiotics
    c. Circumcision is usually required for penile zip entrapment
    d. All hernias in patients younger than 1 year require surgical intervention
    e. Epidymo-orchitis is common in the paediatric population

5.12 Causes of haematuria:

    a. Rifampicin
    b. Exercise
    c. Hypercalciuria
    d. Pyelonephritis
    e. Rhabdomyolysis

5.13 Causes of stridor:

    a. Acute laryngotracheobronchitis
    b. Diphtheria
    c. Bronchiolitis
    d. Laryngomalacia
    e. Asthma

5.14 Causes of purpuric rashes in children:

    a. Trauma
    b. Thrombocytopenia
    c. Kawasaki disease
    d. Erythema marginatum
    e. Erythema toxicum

5.15 Regarding paediatric trauma:

    a. Drowning is the most common traumatic cause of death
    b. Children have a reduced surface area to body weight ratio
    c. Fluid bolus of 10 ml/kg should be administered if required
    d. Hypotension is an early indicator of hypovolaemia
    e. Children have increased susceptibility to hypothermia

5.16 Regarding paediatric trauma:

    a. Shoulder dislocations are common
    b. Significant intrathoracic injuries can occur without rib fractures
    c. Pseudosubluxation of C2 on C3 is a relatively common finding
    d. Cervical spine injuries tend to affect the upper (C1–C3) instead of the lower C spine
    e. Fractures are more common than ligamentous injuries

5.17 Regarding paediatric trauma:

a. A Guedel airway is sized by measuring the distance between the centre of the teeth and the angle of the mandible
b. In cardiac arrest 10 mg/kg of adrenaline should be given
c. A reservoir bag decreases the concentration of oxygen delivered to a patient
d. Internal diameter of the ET tube in mm is (age/2) + 4
e. Oropharyngeal airways should be inserted the 'right way up'

5.18 Regarding paediatric trauma:

a. Children have increased body weight to surface area ratio
b. Rotatory subluxation can cause significant injury without fracture occurring
c. DPL is preferred to CT abdomen
d. Two vomits post head injury indicate serious intracranial pathology
e. Up to 200 μg/kg of morphine may be given to children older than 12 months

5.19 Regarding paediatric medicine:

a. A 7 year old child weighs 22 kg on average
b. Expected SBP in a 2 year old is 84 mmHg
c. Total blood volume is typically 80 ml/kg
d. Femoral lines are contraindicated in children younger than 12 years
e. Meningitis C vaccination is given at 12–15 months

5.20 Regarding the neonatal period:

a. A 1 week old baby requires 50 ml/kg/day oral intake
b. A newborn baby loses up to 10% of his/her birth weight in the first week
c. Jaundice within 24 hours of birth is normal
d. The distal femur may be used for intraosseous access
e. A straight blade laryngoscope is used in neonates

5.21 Regarding upper respiratory chest infections:

a. Croup is worse in the mornings
b. Pertussis vaccination has made epiglottitis a rare condition
c. Nebulized budesonide is used in patients with croup
d. Acute laryngotracheobronchitis is associated with hoarseness
e. Needle cricothyroidotomy is contraindicated in children younger than 12 years

5.22 Causes of abdominal pain in children:

a. Hyperosmolar non-ketotic acidosis
b. Pneumonia
c. Wilm's tumour
d. Migraine
e. Pregnancy

5.23 Regarding renal failure in children:

a. Nephrotic syndrome is usually associated with a recent diarrhoeal illness
b. Nephrotic syndrome is associated with cerebral venous thrombosis
c. Haemolytic uraemic syndrome is associated with encephalopathy
d. Sodium nitroprusside is used to treat renal failure-induced hypertension
e. Post-renal renal failure is the most common type

5.24 Regarding pneumonia in children:

a. *E. coli* is a common cause in neonates
b. Cavitation suggests *Haem. influenzae* as the causative organism
c. Associated headaches suggest mycoplasma as the cause
d. Usually associated with the classic signs of consolidation in children
e. *Strep. pneumoniae* is the most common cause in older children

5.1 Answers

a. **False** – expected to transfer objects at 6 months
b. **False** – able to turn head to sound at 3–4 months
c. **True**
d. **True**
e. **True**

5.2 Answers

a. **True**
b. **True**
c. **False** – PEF < 50% of best or predicted is a feature of acute severe asthma in children older than 5 years
d. **False** – silent chest is a feature of life-threatening asthma
e. **False** – a respiratory rate of 12 breaths/min is a sign of failing respiratory effort

5.3 Answers

a. **False** – often no cause for asthma is found
b. **False** – pulmonary function testing is only used in children older than 7 years due to technique involved
c. **True**
d. **True**
e. **True**

5.4 Answers

a. **False**
b. **False**
c. **True**
d. **False**
e. **True**

5.5 Answers

a. **True** – represents poor coping abilities
b. **True** – preterm infants have an increased risk of apnoea
c. **False** – bronchodilator therapy is not proven to be of benefit
d. **False** – crackles are a common finding; CXR should only be done if suspicion of co-existent chest infection
e. **False**

5.6 Answers

a. **False** – Emla cream contains lignocaine and prilocaine
b. **True**
c. **False**
d. **True**
e. **False**

5.7 Answers

a. **False**
b. **True**
c. **False** – a full history and examination need to be performed to determine what investigations are necessary; the presence of pyrexia does not obviate the need for further tests
d. **True**
e. **False** – according to guidelines patients on regular phenytoin should be commenced on a phenobarbitone infusion as first line

5.8 Answers

a. **False** – IV lorazepam is recommended for treatment
b. **True**
c. **False** – seizures can cause a pyrexia also
d. **True**
e. **False** – recommended that a phenobarbitone infusion be given; phenytoin infusions should be used in patients not on phenytoin

5.9 Answers

a. **False** – as the blockage is proximal to the ampulla of vater
b. **False** – hypertrophic pyloric stenosis is associated with hypochloraemic alkalosis
c. **False** – the child is usually hungry after vomiting
d. **False** – correction of dehydration and electrolyte imbalance is required before surgery
e. **False** – a palpable abdominal mass may be present but not always

5.10 Answers

a. **False** – intussusception is most common between 6 months and 3 years
b. **True** – however, an abdominal mass is not always present
c. **True** – however, patients are not always pain free between episodes
d. **False**
e. **False** – barium enemas are not contraindicated; either barium or air enemas may be used depending on site preferences

5.11 Answers

a. **False** – foreskin is usually retractile by age 5
b. **False** – balanitis is usually managed with oral antibiotics
c. **False** – circumcision is rarely required
d. **False** – infants often outgrow hernias by the age of 1 year
e. **False** – epidymo-orchitis is rare in the paediatric population

5.12 Answers

a. **False** – rifampicin discolours urine but does not actually cause haematuria
b. **True**
c. **True**
d. **True**
e. **False** – rhabdomyolysis causes myoglobinuria which causes a false-positive reading on dipstick analysis

5.13 Answers

a. **True** – acute laryngotracheobronchitis is commonly known as croup
b. **True** – although diphtheria is rare now due to vaccination
c. **False**
d. **True**
e. **False** – stridor is a sign of upper airway obstruction

5.14 Answers

a. **True**
b. **True** – e.g. due to leukaemia, idiopathic thrombocytopenic purpura
c. **False** – Kawasaki disease causes a desquamating rash of the palms of the hands and feet
d. **False** – this erythematous rash is transient and has raised edges. Occurs in approximately 20% of patients with rheumatic fever
e. **False** – erythema toxicum occurs during the first few days of life; the rash is red with central white vesicles

5.15 Answers

a. **False** – drowning is the third most common cause. Road traffic accidents are the most common cause of death, followed by fires
b. **False** – children have an increased surface area to body weight ratio
c. **False** – fluid boluses of 20 ml/kg should be administered
d. **False** – as in the elderly, hypotension is a late sign
e. **True** – hypothermia susceptibility is increased due to a child's high surface area to body weight ratio

5.16 Answers

a. **False** – shoulder dislocations are rare in this age group; common sites for dislocations are the patella or radius (pulled elbows)
b. **True**
c. **True**
d. **True**
e. **True** – fractures are more common due to the relatively soft bones in children

5.17 Answers

a. **True**
b. **False** – 10 μg/kg of adrenaline should be given in cardiac arrest
c. **False** – a reservoir bag increases the concentration of oxygen given
d. **False** – the calculation is (age/4) + 4
e. **True** – oropharyngeal airways should be inserted 'right way up' to avoid pharyngeal trauma

5.18 Answers

a. **False** – children have an increased surface area to body weight ratio
b. **True**
c. **False** – CT abdomen or ultrasound is preferred to DPL
d. **False** – two vomits post head injury can be normal in children
e. **True**

5.19 Answers

a. **True** – weight in kg = (age + 4) x 2
b. **True** – SBP = (age x 2) + 80
c. **True**
d. **False**
e. **False** – meningitis C vaccination is given at 2, 3, and 4 months

5.20 Answers

a. **False** – a 1 week old baby requires 150 ml/kg/day oral intake
b. **True**
c. **False** – jaundice in the first 24 hrs is considered abnormal and requires further investigation
d. **True** – 3 cm above the lower lateral femoral condyle on the anterolateral surface
e. **True**

5.21 Answers

a. **False** – croup is worse at night
b. **False** - Hib vaccination has made epiglottis a rare condition
c. **True**
d. **True**
e. **False** – surgical; needle cricothyroidotomy is contraindicated in children younger than 12 years

5.22 Answers

a. **False** – diabetic ketoacidosis may cause hyperosmolar non-ketotic acidosis
b. **True**
c. **True** – Wilm's tumour is a nephroblastoma
d. **True** – children often have difficulty localizing pain
e. **True** – in adolescents

5.23 Answers

a. **False** – haemolytic uraemic syndrome is associated with a recent diarrhoeal illness
b. **True**
c. **True**
d. **True**
e. **False** – pre-renal and post-renal renal are more common than post-renal failure

5.24 Answers

a. **True**
b. **False** – cavitation is suggestive of TB or staphylococcus infection
c. **True**
d. **False** – classic signs of consolidation are often absent in children
e. **True**

6. Surgery

6.1 Regarding subarachnoid haemorrhage:

    a. Most common cause is trauma
    b. Fundoscopy may show subhyaloid haemorrhages
    c. There is increased incidence in patients with polycystic kidneys and neurofibromatosis
    d. Associated with QT prolongation
    e. Smoking is a risk factor for subarachnoid haemorrhage

6.2 Regarding subarachnoid haemorrhage:

    a. Complications include rebleeding
    b. Complications include cerebral vasospasm – maximum at day 3–15
    c. A negative CT brain rules out a subarachnoid haemorrhage
    d. Lumbar puncture should be performed within 6 hours of onset of symptoms
    e. Nimodipine helps manage cerebral vasospasm

6.3 Regarding haematemesis:

    a. Associated with aortic aneurysm
    b. Associated with raised urea
    c. Associated with burns
    d. It has a poor prognosis in patients with chronic renal failure
    e. Barrett's oesophagus does not affect children

6.4 Regarding upper gastrointestinal haemorrhage:

    a. Gastric ulcers are more common than duodenal ulcers
    b. Meckel's diverticulum is a common cause in patients over 40 years old
    c. Lactulose is used in the management of variceal haemorrhage
    d. Calcium gluconate should be administered with every 3 units of red blood cells transfused
    e. Vasopressin is used in conjunction with metoclopramide in the management of variceal haemorrhages

6.5 Regarding the treatment of upper gastrointestinal haemorrhage:

    a. Diuretics are used in management
    b. Octreotide is used in management
    c. Biphosphonates are used in management
    d. Rivastigmine is used in management
    e. Nitrates are used in duodenal ulcer bleeds

6.6 **Regarding rectal bleeding:**

a. Angiodysplasia predominately affects the right colon and caecum
b. Diverticulosis causes painful pr bleeding
c. Haemorrhoids are the most common cause in patients over 50
d. Acute mesenteric infarction causes painless pr bleeds
e. Management of patients require inpatient investigations

6.7 **Regarding rectal bleeding:**

a. Ischaemic colitis most commonly affects the splenic flexure
b. Ischaemic colitis is associated with thumb printing on abdominal X-ray
c. Ischaemic colitis affects the mucosa and submucosa
d. Always originates distal to the ligament of Treitz
e. Anal fissures are usually located anteriorly and in the midline

6.8 **Regarding aortic aneurysms:**

a. Infrarenal aneurysms have a better prognosis than suprarenal aneurysms
b. The majority of aneurysms are infrarenal
c. Patients with COPD have an increased risk of rupture
d. All ruptures require vigorous IV fluid resuscitation
e. They are associated with neurological deficits

6.9 **Regarding aortic aneurysms:**

a. Increased incidence in first-degree relatives
b. Rupture usually occurs into the right retroperitoneum
c. Rupture risk increases in proportion to the level of hypertension
d. A systolic blood pressure of > 120 mmHg is recommended
e. Most common cause of death is myocardial infarction

6.10 **Regarding aortic aneurysms:**

a. If spinal cord ischaemia occurs it usually affects the lumbar region first
b. Abdominal X-ray to look for calcified aortic aneurysm is recommended in suspected cases
c. Splenic artery aneurysm is more common in females
d. Associated with a risk of salmonella infection
e. Onset of back pain signals an impending rupture

6.11 **Causes of raised amylase:**

a. Acute cholecystitis
b. Mesenteric infarction
c. Renal calculus
d. Mumps
e. Diabetic ketoacidosis

6.12 **Causes of acute pancreatitis:**

   a. Hypocalcaemia
   b. Gastric carcinoma
   c. Cystic fibrosis
   d. Amoxicillin
   e. Hyperthermia

6.13 **Regarding pancreatitis:**

   a. It is associated with Epstein–Barr virus
   b. It is associated with hypercalcaemia
   c. It is associated with hyperparathyroidism
   d. Poor prognosis is associated with a urea of > 7 mmol/L
   e. Poor prognosis is associated with a glucose < 10 mmol/L

6.14 **Regarding pancreatitis:**

   a. Abscess formation is an early complication
   b. Glasgow Scoring Scale (GSS) is performed at admission and at 72 hours
   c. GSS examines LDH and bilirubin levels
   d. GSS examines age, respiratory rate, and blood pressure
   e. May be caused by steroids or diuretic use

6.15 **Regarding obstructive jaundice:**

   a. Causes a prolonged prothrombin time
   b. Sclerosing cholangitis is a cause
   c. Causes a prolonged half-life of morphine
   d. Increases ALP/GGT >> AST/ALT
   e. It is associated with decreased urinary conjugated bilirubin

6.16 **Regarding portal hypertension:**

   a. Refers to portal pressures > 15 mmHg
   b. Pericarditis is a cause of portal hypertension
   c. Cirrhosis is the most common cause in the UK
   d. Child–Pugh classification assesses the type of cirrhosis
   e. Child–Pugh classification assesses bilirubin, albumin, and PT levels

6.17 **Regarding splenectomy:**

   a. Indications include idiopathic thrombocytopenic purpura
   b. Indications include thalassaemia
   c. Indications include hereditary spherocytosis
   d. Indications include malaria
   e. Post-splenectomy complications include thrombophilia

6.18 Regarding bowel obstruction:

a. It is associated with metabolic acidosis
b. It is associated with metabolic alkalosis
c. Large bowel obstruction is more common than small bowel obstruction
d. Severe pain or marked leukocytosis are indicators of strangulation
e. Adhesions are the most common cause of small bowel obstruction

6.19 Regarding bowel obstruction:

a. Barium meal is helpful to aid diagnosis
b. Antibiotic prophylaxis against sepsis is not indicated
c. A ' closed loop' radiologically is an indication for immediate surgery
d. Feculent vomiting is a feature of small bowel obstruction
e. Small bowel obstruction is most commonly secondary to neoplastic lesions

6.20 Regarding inflammatory bowel disease:

a. It is associated with pyoderma gangrenosum
b. Ulcerative colitis is associated with sclerosing cholangitis
c. Crohn's disease is associated with granulomas
d. Ulcerative colitis is associated with increased incidence of cholelithiasis and nephrolithiasis
e. Most common site for Crohn's disease is the ileocolonic region

6.21 Causes of recurrent perianal abscesses:

a. Inflammatory bowel disease
b. Colonic carcinoma
c. Diabetes mellitus
d. Steroids
e. Colonic polyps

6.22 Regarding acute epididymo-orchitis:

a. It is associated with infertility
b. Pain is relieved by elevating the testis
c. N. gonorrhea is a common bacterial cause
d. Associated with testicular infarction
e. All patients should have antibiotic therapy

6.23 Regarding testicular torsion:

a. A non-viable testis should always be removed
b. Usually presents with abdominal pain and vomiting post trauma
c. Most common in teenagers
d. Does not always require urgent referral
e. Opposite testis lies horizontal not vertical

6.24   Signs of arterial ischaemia:

   a. Rest pain
   b. Red discolouration of the lower limb
   c. Limp
   d. Lateral leg ulceration
   e. ABPI 1.2

6.25   Regarding malignant hyperthermia:

   a. It is an autosomal dominant condition
   b. It may be induced by the use of halothane
   c. It is associated with supraventricular tachycardias
   d. It is associated with hypokalaemia
   e. Procainamide is used in management

6.1 Answers

a. **True**
b. **True**
c. **True**
d. **True**
e. **True**

6.2 Answers

a. **True** – 10% of subarachnoid haemorrhages rebleed within hours, 30% within 4 weeks, and 50% within 6 months
b. **True**
c. **False** – up to 5% of subarachnoid haemorrhages may be missed on CT
d. **False** – lumbar puncture examines for the presence of the breakdown products of haemoglobin which require at least 6 hours to be seen
e. **True** – nimodipine is a calcium channel antagonist

6.3 Answers

a. **True** – from an aortoenteric fistula, often post repair of an aortic aneurysm
b. **True** – due to the increased protein load in the gut and co-existent hypovolaemia
c. **True** – from stress ulceration
d. **True** – co-morbidities increase the death rate
e. **False** – Barrett's oesophagus is rarely congenital in origin and seen in children as young as 2 years

6.4 Answers

a. **False** – duodenal ulcers are more common than gastric ulcers
b. **False** – Meckel's diverticulum is rare in patients over 25 years old
c. **True** – lactulose is used to prevent hepatic encephalopathy
d. **True** – calcium levels decrease post multiple transfusions due to citrate metabolism
e. **True** – vasopressin causes splanchnic vasoconstriction and metoclopramide increases lower oesophageal pressure and decreases azygous blood flow

6.5 Answers

a. **False** – diuretics would worsen hypovolaemia
b. **True** – octreotide is a synthetic analogue of somatostatin and lacks the peripheral side-effects of vasopressin
c. **False**
d. **False** – rivastigmine is a cholinesterase inhibitor
e. **False** – nitrates are used for variceal haemorrhages; in conjunction with vasopressin they decrease the peripheral side-effects and augment the reduction of portal pressure

6.6 Answers

a. **True**
b. **False** – diverticulosis usually causes painless pr bleeds
c. **False** – haemorrhoids are the most common cause in the under 50 year age group.
d. **False** – acute mesenteric infarction usually causes painful pr bleeds
e. **False** – many patients can be managed on an outpatient basis

6.7 Answers

a. **True**
b. **True**
c. **True**
d. **False** – 10–15% of rectal bleeds originate proximal to the ligament of Treitz
e. **False** – anal fissures are usually located posteriorly and in the midline

6.8 Answers

a. **True**
b. **True**
c. **True**
d. **False** – vigorous IV fluid resuscitation risks losing tamponade effect. Only needed if hypovolaemic arrest, very hypotensive, or ischaemic organ failure. Aim for systolic blood pressure of 80–100 mmHg
e. **True** – due to spinal cord ischaemia

6.9 Answers

a. **True**
b. **False** – aortic aneurysms usually bleed into the left retroperitoneum
c. **True**
d. **False** – an SBP of 80–100 mmHg is recommended to prevent rupture of a tamponade
e. **False** – hypotension-induced multiorgan failure is the most common cause of death

6.10 Answers

a. **False** – spinal cord ischaemia usually affects the T10–T12 region first
b. **False** – abdominal X-ray is not a sensitive test
c. **True** – splenic artery aneurysm is thought to be more common in females owing to the effect of oestrogen on the arterial wall
d. **True** – blood-borne organisms may infect clefts in the thrombus; salmonella and *Staph. aureus* are the most commonly implicated organisms
e. **True**

6.11 Answers

a. **True**
b. **True**
c. **False**
d. **True**
e. **True**

6.12 Answers

a. **False** – hypercalcaemia is a cause
b. **False** – pancreatic carcinoma is the cause in up to 3% of cases
c. **True**
d. **False**
e. **False** – hypothermia is associated with acute pancreatitis

6.13 Answers

a. **True** – pancreatitis is associated with infectious mononucleosis
b. **False** – pancreatitis is associated with hypocalcaemia
c. **False** – pancreatitis is associated with hyperparathyroidism
d. **False** – urea levels > 16 mmol/L are associated with a poor prognosis
e. **False** – glucose levels > 10 mmol/L are associated with a poor prognosis

6.14 Answers

a. **False** – abscess formation is a late complication
b. **False** – GSS is performed at admission and 48 hours
c. **False** – bilirubin is not considered; LDH and AST are assessed
d. **False** – of these only age is considered
e. **True**

6.15 Answers

a. **True**
b. **True**
c. **True**
d. **True**
e. **False** – obstructive jaundice is associated with increased urinary conjugated bilirubin

6.16 Answers

a. **False** – portal hypertension refers to portal pressures > 12 mmHg
b. **True** – constrictive pericarditis causes post-hepatic portal hypertension
c. **True**
d. **False** – the Child–Pugh classification assesses the severity of cirrhosis
e. **True**

6.17 Answers

a. **True**
b. **True**
c. **True**
d. **True** – if malaria causes a haemolytic anaemia
e. **True**

6.18 Answers

a. **True** – if severe vomiting is present
b. **True** – if the patient becomes shocked or dehydrated
c. **False**
d. **True**
e. **True**

6.19 Answers

a. **False** – barium meal is contraindicated
b. **False** – antibiotic prophylaxis against sepsis should be considered
c. **True** – immediate surgery is indicated because of the risk of bowel ischaemia and perforation
d. **False** – feculent vomiting is a sign of large bowel obstruction
e. **False** – adhesions and incarcerated hernias are the most common causes of small bowel obstruction

6.20 Answers

a. **True**
b. **True**
c. **True**
d. **False**
e. **True**

6.21 Answers

a. **True**
b. **True**
c. **True**
d. **True**
e. **False**

6.22 Answers

a. **True**
b. **True**
c. **True**
d. **True**
e. **False** – antibiotic therapy would not be of benefit to patients with viral- or drug-induced epididymorchitis

6.23 Answers

a. **True** – as antibodies will cause infertility
b. **True**
c. **True** – 12–22 years is the most common age group for testicular torsion
d. **False** – delay may cause a nonviable testis
e. **True** – Angell's sign

6.24 Answers

a. **True** – rest pain occurs at night due to a fall in blood flow below that needed for tissue metabolism
b. **True** – red discolouration of the lower limb occurs in advanced stages due to capillary blood stasis and high O_2 demand
c. **True** – limp is a sign of claudication
d. **True**
e. **False** – normal >1; < 0.92 indicates arterial disease, and 0.5–< 0.9 indicates claudication

6.25 Answers

a. **True**
b. **True**
c. **True**
d. **False** – malignant hyperthermia is associated with hyperkalaemia
e. **True** – procainamide increases calcium uptake and helps prevent ventricular arrhythmias

7. Infectious diseases

7.1 Regarding meningitis:

a. Coagulopathy is not a contraindication to lumbar puncture
b. Dexamethasone is recommended for *Haem. influenzae* type B meningitis
c. CSF glucose < 2.2 mmol/L and CSF protein > 2 g/L indicate bacterial meningitis
d. Otitis media is a recognized risk factor
e. Group B Strep. is a common causative organism in the neonatal period

7.2 The following CSF findings are consistent with a bacterial meningitis:

a. Protein 3 g/L
b. Glucose 2.5 mmol/L
c. WCC < 500/–l
d. Glucose CSF:serum ratio of 0.2
e. CSF pressure 40 mmHg

7.3 Regarding meningitis:

a. Associated with adrenal haemorrhage
b. Viral meningitis has a poorer prognosis than bacterial meningitis
c. Lumbar puncture should be performed in all suspected cases
d. TB meningitis usually has a rapid clinical onset
e. All hospital staff in contact with the patient require prophylaxis

7.4 Infectious mononucleosis is associated with:

a. Beta-haemolytic strep. infection
b. Splenic rupture
c. Pancreatitis
d. Jaundice
e. Facial palsy

7.5 Regarding infectious hepatitis:

a. Patients are maximally infectious before the onset of jaundice
b. Hepatitis B is the most common blood–borne virus in the UK
c. Hepatitis A is transmitted via the faecal–oral route
d. Hepatitis D requires the presence of hepatitis C to replicate
e. Both hepatitis C and hepatitis B are associated with increased risk of hepatocellular carcinoma

7.6   **Regarding rabies:**

   a. It is a viral infection
   b. It is associated with hydrophobia
   c. Immunization is available
   d. Death is usually secondary to aspiration pneumonia
   e. Infection may occur post bite or inhalation

7.7   **Regarding severe acute respiratory syndrome (SARS):**

   a. Caused by an RNA retrovirus
   b. Spread by the faecal–oral route
   c. WCC is usually significantly increased
   d. Nebulizers are used in treatment
   e. Oxygen should be administered at a rate of < 6 L/min

7.8   **Regarding HIV infection:**

   a. It is an RNA retrovirus
   b. A CD4 count $< 400/\text{mm}^3$ is defined as AIDS
   c. Patients with STDs have increased risk of transmission during unprotected intercourse
   d. In at-risk patients HIV testing should be performed in A&E
   e. Pregnant staff can safely treat patients with AIDS

7.9   **Regarding HIV infection:**

   a. In PCP pneumonia CXR typically shows infiltrates in bilateral upper zones
   b. CMV retinitis causes painful reduced visual acuity
   c. CMV retinitis is associated with perivascular haemorrhage and exudate on fundoscopy
   d. Kaposi's sarcoma can cause dysphagia
   e. Patients with AIDS have an increased incidence of salmonella septicaemia

7.10   **Regarding hepatitis:**

   a. Hepatitis A is spread via the blood-borne route
   b. Hepatitis A is associated with tender hepatomegaly
   c. The majority of patients with hepatitis B fully recover
   d. It is associated with glomerulonephritis
   e. Hepatitis C can be transmitted from shared heroin cooking equipment

7.11   **Regarding anthrax:**

   a. Airborne transmission from person to person occurs
   b. Cutaneous anthrax causes painful ulceration
   c. Diagnosis is made by urinalysis
   d. Pulmonary anthrax is more common than cutaneous anthrax
   e. It is a notifiable disease in the UK

7.12 **Septic arthritis:**

    a. Patients with sickle cell disease have increased incidence of salmonella septic arthritis
    b. *Staph. aureus* is a common pathogen
    c. Chronic arthritis is a recognized risk factor
    d. Joint drainage is recommended after antibiotic therapy
    e. *Neisseira gonorrhea* infection is most common in the neonatal period

7.13 **Regarding tonsillitis:**

    a. Tonsillitis should be treated with co-amoxiclav if there is a history of immunosuppression
    b. Quinsy causes uvula deviation away from the affected side
    c. Group A beta-haemolytic streptococci is the most common cause of bacterial tonsillitis
    d. Presence of pus on the tonsils confirms the presence of a bacterial tonsillitis
    e. Splenomegaly indicates a viral aetiology

7.14 **Regarding incubation time:**

    a. Hepatitis A = 3–4 weeks
    b. Salmonella enteritis = 48–72 hours
    c. Tetanus = 4–14 days
    d. Mumps = 14–18 days
    e. Rabies = 3–12 weeks

7.15 **Regarding infectious mononucleosis:**

    a. Average incubation period is 4–6 weeks
    b. The sore throat typically lasts for 5 days
    c. Treated with steroids
    d. All patients are monospot positive
    e. Up to 5% of cases are caused by cytomegalovirus

7.1 Answers

a. **False**
b. **True** – dexamethasone reduces the incidence of long-term complications in children, such as sensorineural deafness or recurrent seizures
c. **True**
d. **True**
e. **True**

7.2 Answers

a. **True**
b. **False** – glucose < 2.2 would be consistent with a bacterial meningitis
c. **False** – a WCC > 500 would be consistent with a bacterial meningitis
d. **True**
e. **True**

7.3 Answers

a. **True** – Waterhouse–Friderichsen syndrome
b. **False**
c. **False** – lumbar puncture should not be performed if there is a contraindication such as coagulopathy
d. **False** – TB meningitis often has a slow insidious onset
e. **False** – hospital staff only require prophylaxis if they perform mouth-to-mouth resuscitation

7.4 Answers

a. **True** – up to 25% of patients have co-infection with beta-haemolytic strep.
b. **True**
c. **True**
d. **True**
e. **True**

7.5 Answers

a. **True**
b. **False** – hepatitis C is the most common blood–borne virus in the UK
c. **True**
d. **False** – hepatitis D requires the presence of hepatitis B to replicate
e. **True**

7.6 Answers

a. **True**
b. **True**
c. **True**
d. **False** – death is usually secondary to paralysis
e. **True** – infection rarely occurs post inhalation

7.7 Answers

a. **False** – SARS is caused by a cornovirus
b. **False** – SARS is transmitted by the respiratory route
c. **False** – WCC is often normal initially
d. **False** – nebulizers increase the risk of SARS transmission; space inhalers should be used instead
e. **True** – to avoid aerolization of the virus

7.8 Answers

a. **True**
b. **False** – CD4 counts < 200/mm^3 are defined as AIDS
c. **True** – patients with STDs have increased incidence of mucosal breaches
d. **False** – HIV testing should be arranged in an infectious disease clinic with counselling facilities
e. **False** – it is unsafe for pregnant staff to treat patients with AIDS due to the risk of herpes simplex infection and cytomegalovirus infection

7.9 Answers

a. **False** – typically bilateral midzone infiltrates are present on CXR
b. **True**
c. **True**
d. **True**
e. **True**

7.10 Answers

a. **False** – hepatitis A is spread via the faecal–oral route
b. **True**
c. **True**
d. **True**
e. **True** – this is important information to convey to IV drug abusers

7.11 Answers

a. **False** – airborne transmission only occurs via spores, not person to person
b. **False** – cutaneous anthrax causes a painless ulceration
c. **False** – diagnosis is made by MC&S of a pustule
d. **False** – pulmonary anthrax is more serious than cutaneous anthrax
e. **True**

7.12 Answers

a. **True**
b. **True**
c. **True**
d. **False** – joint drainage is recommended before antibiotic treatment to allow cultures to be taken
e. **False** – *Neisseira gonorrhea* infection is common in young adults

7.13 Answers

a. **False** – co-amoxiclav causes a rash if Epstein–Barr virus is present
b. **True**
c. **True**
d. **False** – the presence of pus suggests bacterial tonsillitis but is not diagnostic
e. **True** – occurs with Epstein–Barr virus (glandular fever)

7.14 Answers

a. **True**
b. **False** – 6–48 hours
c. **True**
d. **True**
e. **True**

7.15 Answers

a. **True**
b. **False** – the sore throat usually lasts 7 days at least
c. **True** – steroids are used in cases of anginose infectious mononucleosis or in patients with neurological complications
d. **False** – up to 80% of patients are monospot positive
e. **False** – infectious mononucleosis is caused by Epstein-Barr virus

8. Specialties

8.1 **Regarding statistical terms:**

    a. Specificity is the term used to describe the precision associated with the estimate of the mean

    b. Sensitivity refers to the true-positive ratio; that is the proportion of patients with disease who return a positive test

    c. Standard deviation refers to the measure of the spread of a distribution and is equal to the square root of the variance

    d. In a frequency distribution the mode is the most frequently observed value

    e. If a measurement has a skewed distribution, then the mean and the mode are always different

8.2 **Regarding statistical terms:**

    a. Annual prevalence of a condition reflects the number of new cases reported annually

    b. Standard deviation of a population may be smaller than the standard error of a sample mean from that population

    c. Median is the point on a scale of values which exactly divides the number of values into upper and lower halves

    d. In a frequency distribution the mode is the most frequently observed value

    e. $P = 0.01$ is a lower degree of statistical significance than $P = 0.05$

8.3 **Regarding statistical terms:**

    a. Standard deviation is the square of the variance of the group

    b. Standard deviation may be used as a basis for the calculation of the chi-squared value

    c. Standard deviation is the measure of a scatter of the observations around the mean

    d. In a type 1 error the null hypothesis is wrongly rejected

    e. The null hypothesis is true if there are significant differences between the response of the treatment and placebo groups

8.4 **In a normal (Gaussian) distribution:**

    a. The mode is the most frequently observed value

    b. All the people in the sample are normal

    c. Mean, mode, and median are numerically the same

    d. Median divides the distribution exactly into two halves

    e. Distribution is numerically the same as a Poisson distribution

8.5   Suicide risk factors:

a. Female sex
b. Unemployed
c. Passive thoughts about being harmed
d. Recent self-harm
e. Severity of depression

8.6   Regarding suicide:

a. Unemployed people are more at risk than those in stressful jobs
b. Patients with chronic physical illness have increased risk
c. Recent bereavement increases risk
d. Most common in young women
e. It is associated with alcohol abuse

8.7   Suicide risk factors:

a. Active plans
b. Schizophrenia
c. Elderly
d. Divorce
e. Job promotion

8.8   The following are recognized complications of diabetes in pregnancy:

a. Pre-eclampsia
b. Congenital abnormalities
c. Intrauterine growth retardation
d. Polyhydramnios
e. Respiratory distress in the newborn

8.9   Regarding pre-eclampsia:

a. Increased risk during first pregnancy
b. Increased risk if carrying twins
c. Associated with DIC
d. Associated with thrombophilia
e. Hypertension is controlled with ACE inhibitors

8.10 Regarding the post-partum period:

a. Pelvic infection risk is increased by repeated vaginal examination
b. Symptoms of infection include uterine subinvolution and yellow lochia
c. Co-amoxiclav may be taken while breastfeeding
d. Retained products of conception cause increased risk of primary and secondary post-partum haemorrhage
e. Pelvic infection causes an increased risk of pulmonary embolus

8.11 Drugs contraindicated while breastfeeding:

a. Lithium
b. Aspirin
c. ACE inhibitors
d. Sulphonamides
e. Paracetamol

8.12 Regarding ectopic pregnancy:

a. Endometriosis increases the risk
b. It is always associated with vaginal bleeding
c. Does not occur after tubal ligation
d. Uterine horn implantation is relatively safe
e. Is the largest cause of maternal mortality in the second trimester

8.13 Regarding vaginal bleeding:

a. Trophoblastic disease most commonly causes bleeding after 20 weeks' gestation
b. Increased parity is a risk factor for abruptio placenta
c. Abruptio placenta is a recognized risk factor for DIC
d. Placenta praevia causes painful vaginal bleeding
e. All patients with vaginal bleeding should have a vaginal examination

8.14 Regarding miscarriage:

a. Maternal age older than 30 increases the risk of spontaneous abortion
b. Retained products post 'miscarriage' should be electively removed
c. Cervical shock refers to a dilated cervix and severe bleeding
d. All patients post miscarriage should receive 500 mg of ergometrine
e. All Rhesus-positive patients with vaginal bleeding should receive 250 units of anti-D immunoglobulin

8.15 Regarding emergency contraception:

a. Intrauterine contraceptive devices should be placed within 5 days of intercourse
b. Patients with pelvic inflammatory disease can have intrauterine contraceptive devices safely inserted
c. Risk of pregnancy is greatest if the oral contraceptive pill is missed in the last 7 days of the menstrual cycle
d. Breastfeeding is a contraindication for the 'morning after' pill
e. Epilepsy is a contraindication for the 'morning after' pill

8.16 **Cataracts are associated with:**

 a. Thyrotoxicosis
 b. Rubella
 c. Hyperparathyroidism
 d. Myotonic dystrophy
 e. Paget's disease

8.17 **Regarding visual loss:**

 a. Quinine overdose causes a loss of vision
 b. Giant cell arteritis affects the posterior ciliary arteries
 c. IV acetazolamide is used to reduce intraocular pressure
 d. Acute glaucoma causes a fixed pupil
 e. There is an increased incidence of glaucoma in hypermetropic patients

8.18 **Regarding retinal detachment:**

 a. Increased incidence in people with myopia
 b. Associated with premonitory flashing lights
 c. Increased incidence in diabetics
 d. Associated with a painful red eye
 e. Is excluded by normal findings on fundoscopy

8.19 **Red eye is associated with:**

 a. Acute iritis
 b. Central retinal vein occlusion
 c. Optic neuritis
 d. Ulcerative keratitis
 e. Ectropion

8.20 **Painless loss of vision is associated with:**

 a. Central retinal artery occlusion
 b. Vitreous haemorrhage
 c. Optic neuritis
 d. Blepharitis
 e. Acute closed angle glaucoma

8.21 **Regarding altitude illness:**

 a. Dexamethasone is contraindicated
 b. Diuretics are used in management
 c. Acetazolamide is used in management
 d. Noncardiogenic pulmonary oedema usually occurs within 12 hours of ascent
 e. Respiratory acidosis occurs

8.22 **Regarding radiation accidents:**

   a. Associated with increased lymphocyte counts
   b. Initial symptoms include nausea, vomiting and diarrhoea
   c. External irradiation has a worse prognosis than contamination with radioactive material
   d. Air conditioning units in the area should be turned off
   e. There may be a latent period between the initial symptoms and the main effects of radiation

8.23 **Regarding dental emergencies:**

   a. Avulsed primary teeth are suitable for re-implantation
   b. Valvular heart disease is a contraindication to re-implantation
   c. Patients with teeth 'missing' after trauma should have a CXR
   d. 0.9% saline should be used to clean avulsed teeth
   e. Patients with toothache should be referred to a maxillofacial surgeon

8.24 **Regarding diving:**

   a. Face mask 'squeeze' commonly is associated with failure to exhale nasally
   b. Aspirin is often used in management of face mask 'squeeze'
   c. Elbows and shoulders are often affected in decompression illness
   d. Patients with decompression illness should be treated with recompression
   e. Decompression illness is associated with peau d'orange skin discolouration

8.25 **Regarding diving:**

   a. Pulmonary barotrauma may cause decompression illness
   b. If an endotracheal tube is used the balloon should be inflated with oxygen
   c. Mediastinal emphysema occurs with ascent barotrauma
   d. If air transporting a patient their diving buddy should be co-transported
   e. If air transporting a patient the plane should fly at between 300 and 500 metres

8.26 **Regarding electrical injury:**

   a. Moisture decreases resistance to flow
   b. Alternate current is less associated with tetany than direct current
   c. Metabolic acidosis is associated
   d. Muscle tissue has higher resistance than fat
   e. Associated with kaerunoparalysis

8.27 **Regarding electrical injury:**

a. Causes myoglobinuria
b. Causes hypokalaemia
c. Causes severe dehydration
d. Associated with late onset of seizure disorders
e. Causes haematuria

8.28 **Regarding heat illness:**

a. Heat stroke is associated with temperatures > 43 °C
b. Active cooling methods should aim for a temperature loss of 1 °C/min
c. It is aggravated by diuretics and salicylates
d. Causes thrombocytopenia and DIC
e. Heat exhaustion occurs before heat cramps

8.29 **Regarding frostbite:**

a. Smoking is a poor prognostic factor
b. Early debridement of wounds is recommended
c. Circulating water of 40 °C is used in management
d. Early exercise is recommended for treatment of local wounds
e. It is defined as tissue freezing due to intracellular ice crystal formation

8.30 **Regarding hypothermia:**

a. Pleural lavage is an example of core exogenous heating
b. Forced air blankets are an example of core exogenous heating
c. Phenothiazines predispose to hypothermia
d. External exogenous rewarming is used for temperatures of 32.5 °C
e. Hypothyroidism and adrenal suppression predispose to hypothermia

8.31 **Regarding hypothermia:**

a. Associated with U waves on ECG
b. Associated with delta waves on ECG
c. Defined as a core temperature of < 33 °C
d. Insulin works effectively at temperatures of 29 °C
e. Arrhythmias become increasingly common once temperatures drop below 30 °C

8.32 **Regarding hypothermia:**

a. Rectal temperature lags behind core temperature
b. It is associated with a raised amylase
c. Parkinson's disease is a risk factor for hypothermia
d. Ventricular fibrillation occurs spontaneously at temperatures < 28 °C
e. Is associated with shortening of the QRS complexes on ECG

8.33 **Regarding near drowning:**

    a. Fresh water has a poorer prognosis than salt water
    b. Asystole has a poor prognosis
    c. Submersion for less than 10 minutes has a good prognosis
    d. Antiarrhythmic treatment should be initiated after rewarming
    e. A first spontaneous breath in under 30 minutes is associated with a good prognosis

8.34 **Regarding burns:**

    a. Parkland burns resuscitation formula should be used for burns of > 7% surface area
    b. Parkland burns resuscitation formula uses 50% normal saline and 50% dextrose as its resuscitation fluid
    c. Parkland burns resuscitation formula calculates resuscitation fluid volume using the formula: 2 ml/kg/% burns area
    d. Muir–Barclay formula use plasma as its resuscitation fluid of choice
    e. If pyrexial the patient may require an extra 10% fluid resuscitation per degree rise in temperature

8.35 **Regarding burns:**

    a. Third-degree burns are painful
    b. All full thickness burns of > 5% should be referred to a burns unit
    c. Patients with rhabdomyolysis require extra fluid replacement
    d. A urine output of 30 ml/kg/h is recommended for adults
    e. CO levels should be checked in patients with carbonaceous sputum

8.36 **Regarding burns:**

    a. Associated with cataracts
    b. Associated with compartment syndrome
    c. Lightning causes a direct current shock
    d. Is low risk to the fetus
    e. Electrical flash burns are deeper than electrical arcing burns

8.37 **Regarding burns:**

    a. Wet cement causes burns through its acid content
    b. Patients with burns > 5% of total body surface area should be given 'prophylactic' antibiotics
    c. Hoarseness is a sign of airway burns
    d. According to the rule of 9s each leg is equal to 9%
    e. Glove and stocking burns in children are a sign of NAI

8.38 Regarding NSAID side-effects:

a. Hypocalcaemia
b. Hyperkalaemia
c. Polycythaemia
d. Haemolytic anaemia
e. Thrombocytopenia

8.39 Regarding acids and alkalis:

a. Acids cause a liquefactive necrosis
b. Acids penetrate tissues deeper than alkalis
c. Alkali ingestion is associated with oesophageal cancer
d. All patients with corrosive ingestions should receive prophylactic antibiotics
e. The pylorus and cricopharyngeus are high risk areas for corrosive ingestion

8.1 Answers

a. **False** – this describes the standard error of the mean
b. **True**
c. **True**
d. **True**
e. **True**

8.2 Answers

a. **False** – the prevalence of a condition reflects the total number of cases in a population at a given time
b. **False** – the standard error of the mean is calculated by dividing the standard deviation of the sample by the square root of the sample size
c. **True**
d. **True**
e. **False** – $P = 0.01$ means the results could have occurred by chance in 1 in a 100 observations, and $P = 0.05$ 1 in 20 observations

8.3 Answers

a. **False** – the standard deviation is the square root of the variance
b. **False** – the chi-squared test is a non-parametric test and is carried out on absolute numbers
c. **True**
d. **True**
e. **False** – the null hypothesis is rejected if there are significant differences between the two groups

8.4 Answers

a. **True**
b. **True**
c. **True**
d. **True**
e. **False** – a Poisson distribution refers to the number of events occurring in a fixed time interval

8.5 Answers

a. **False** – men have higher rates of suicide
b. **True**
c. **False**
d. **True**
e. **True**

8.6 Answers

a. **True**
b. **True** – especially those with chronic painful conditions
c. **True**
d. **False** – most common in young men
e. **True**

8.7 Answers

a. **True**
b. **True**
c. **True**
d. **True**
e. **False**

8.8 Answers

a. **True**
b. **True** – four-fold increased risk of congenital abnormalities
c. **False** – associated with large-for-dates babies; insulin has a growth hormone-like effect on the fetus
d. **True**
e. **True** – the lungs are immature with poor production of surfactant; cortisol is important for lung maturation and is reduced in diabetes

8.9 Answers

a. **True**
b. **True**
c. **True**
False d. **True** – in HELLP syndrome (↓ *platelets*)
e. **False** – ACE inhibitors are harmful to the fetus and are contraindicated

8.10 Answers

a. **True**
b. **False** – the lochia is offensive and discoloured
c. **True**
d. **True**
e. **True** – increased risk of septic pulmonary embolus

8.11 Answers

a. **True** – lithium causes decreased tone and cyanosis
b. **True** – aspirin may cause Reye's syndrome and platelet dysfunction
c. **True**
d. **True** – sulphonamides cause prolonged jaundice
e. **False**

8.12 Answers

a. **True**
b. **False** – intraperitoneal ectopic pregnancy is not associated with vaginal bleeding
c. **False** – there remains a 1 in 6 chance after tubal ligation
d. **False** – uterine horn implantation can reach 10–14 weeks' gestation before rupturing
e. **False** – ectopic pregnancy is the largest cause of maternal mortality in the first trimester

8.13 Answers

a. **False** – trophoblastic disease usually causes bleeding at 10–16 weeks' gestation
b. **True**
c. **True**
d. **False** – placenta praevia usually causes painless vaginal bleeding
e. **False** – patients with vaginal bleeding should not be given a vaginal examination if placenta praevia is suspected

8.14 Answers

a. **True**
b. **False** – retained products should be urgently removed due to the risk of DIC
c. **False** – cervical shock refers to the retained products of conception in the cervical os
d. **False** – ergometrine should only be given if severe bleeding has occurred
e. **False** – Rhesus-negative patients should receive anti-D immunoglobulin

8.15 Answers

a. **True**
b. **False** – pelvic inflammatory disease is a contraindication
c. **False** – the risk of pregnancy is greatest during the first 7 days of the menstrual cycle
d. **True** – due to the risk of oestrogen from the 'morning after' pill passing into the breast milk
e. **False** – although if on hormone-inducing antiepileptics, the dose of the contraceptive pill should be increased by 50%

8.16 Answers

a. **False**
b. **True** – if infected with rubella during pregnancy
c. **True**
d. **True**
e. **False**

8.17 Answers

a. **True**
b. **True**
c. **True**
d. **True**
e. **True**

8.18 Answers

a. **True**
b. **True**
c. **True**
d. **False**
e. **False** – small detachments are often missed on standard fundoscopy

8.19 Answers

a. **True**
b. **False**
c. **False**
d. **True**
e. **False**

8.20 Answers

a. **True**
b. **True**
c. **False** – pain with optic neuritis may be present on eye movement
d. **False** – blepharitis is not associated with loss of vision
e. **False** – acute closed angle glaucoma causes a painful loss of vision

8.21 Answers

a. **False** – dexamethasone is used in the treatment of high altitude encephalopathy
b. **False** – diuretics are not used acutely in the management of altitude illness
c. **True** – prophylactically acetazolamide decreases the incidence and severity of illness
d. **False** – noncardiogenic pulmonary oedema is usually seen at 12–96 days
e. **False** – a mild respiratory alkalosis and hypoxia are seen

8.22 Answers

a. **False** – the lymphocyte counts fall
b. **True**
c. **False**
d. **True**
e. **True**

8.23 Answers

a. **False**
b. **True**
c. **True** – AP and lateral CXR should be taken to exclude the presence of inhaled teeth
d. **True**
e. **False** – only if associated with swelling, trismus, dysphagia, or systemic infection

8.24 Answers

a. **True**
b. **True** – aspirin is used to prevent capillary sludging
c. **True**
d. **True**
e. **True**

8.25 Answers

a. **True** – if pulmonary barotrauma causes release of air bubbles into the pulmonary capillaries
b. **False** – water should be used to inflate the balloon or else it would deflate during recompression treatment
c. **True**
d. **True** – as the diving buddy is at risk also
e. **False** – flights should travel at under 300 metres

8.26 Answers

a. **True**
b. **False**
c. **True** – a lactate acidosis is associated with electrical injury
d. **True**
e. **True** – kaerunoparalysis after lightning injury

8.27 Answers

a. **True**
b. **True**
c. **True** – severe dehydration is due to rapid volume loss into the destroyed or injured tissue
d. **True**
e. **True**

8.28 Answers

a. **False** – heat stroke is associated with temperatures > 41 °C
b. **False** – active cooling methods aim for a temperature loss of 0.1 °C/min
c. **True**
d. **True**
e. **False** – cramps occur at temperatures between 37 and 39 °C; heat exhaustion occurs at temp < 40 °C

8.29 Answers

a. **True** – smoking causes vasoconstriction
b. **False** – early debridement is not recommended unless the wound is septic
c. **True**
d. **False** – the patient should rest until the oedema resolves
e. **True**

8.30 Answers

a. **True**
b. **False** – forced air blankets are an example of external exogenous heating
c. **True** – phenothiazines impair shivering
d. **False** – endogenous rewarming is recommended for temperatures of 32.5 °C
e. **True**

8.31 Answers

a. **False** – U waves on ECG are a sign of hypokalaemia
b. **False** – delta waves on ECG are associated with WPW syndrome
c. **False** – hypothermia is defined as a core temperature of < 35 °C
d. **False** – insulin stops working at temperatures < 30 °C
e. **True**

8.32 Answers

a. **True**
b. **True**
c. **True** – due to immobility
d. **True**
e. **False** – hypothermia is associated with prolonged QRS complexes

8.33 Answers

a. **True**
b. **True**
c. **False** – submersions of < 5 minutes are associated with a good prognosis
d. **True**
e. **True**

8.34 Answers

a. **False** – Parkland burns resuscitation formula should be used in burns of > 10% total body surface area
b. **True**
c. **False** – 4 ml/kg/% burns area is the formula used
d. **True**
e. **True**

8.35 Answers

a. **False** – by definition third-degree burns are painless
b. **True**
c. **True**
d. **True**
e. **True** – as carbonaeceous sputum is a sign of inhalation

8.36 Answers

a. True

b. True – myonecrosis and oedema of muscles may produce compartment syndrome

c. True

d. False – burns are a high risk to the fetus; spontaneous abortion has been reported

e. False – electrical arcing causes deeper burns

8.37 Answers

a. False – the alkali content of wet cement causes burns

b. False

c. True

d. False – each leg is worth 18%

e. True – glove and stocking burns imply forced immersion in hot water

8.38 Answers

a. True

b. True

c. False

d. True

e. True

8.39 Answers

a. False – alkalis cause liquefactive necrosis; acids cause a coagulative necrosis

b. False

c. True

d. False – prophylactic antibiotics have not been proven to be of benefit

e. True

9. Anatomy

9.1 Regarding the anatomy of the anatomical snuffbox:

    a. Contains the scaphoid bone
    b. Contains the trapezium
    c. The radial artery traverses this space
    d. Extensor pollicis brevis lies anteriorly
    e. Extensor pollicis longus lies posteriorly

9.2 Regarding the carpal tunnel:

    a. Runs between the carpal bones and flexor retinaculum
    b. Contains the ulnar nerve
    c. Contains the ulnar artery
    d. Contains the flexor carpi radialis
    e. Contains the tendons of flexor digitorum profundus

9.3 Regarding the brachial plexus:

    a. Radial nerve is derived from the posterior cord
    b. Musculoskeletal nerve supplies the elbow joint flexors
    c. Ulnar nerve is derived from the medial cord
    d. Roots of the brachial plexus run anterior to the scalenus medius
    e. Trunks of the brachial plexus lie at the base of the anterior triangle

9.4 Regarding the hip joint:

    a. Pectineus flexes the thigh
    b. Sartorius medially rotates the thigh at the hip joint
    c. Psoas major medially rotates the thigh
    d. Rectus femoris extends the thigh at the hip joint
    e. Rectus femoris is innervated by the sciatic nerve

9.5 Regarding the hip joint:

    a. Gluteus medius abducts and medially rotates the thigh
    b. Gluteus maximus extends and laterally rotates the thigh
    c. Gluteus maximus is innervated by the superior gluteal nerve
    d. Piriformis helps stabilize the hip joint
    e. Quadriceps muscle group is innervated by the femoral nerve

9.6 **Regarding the popliteal fossa:**

a. Biceps femoris forms the lateral border
b. Tibial nerve lies deep to the popliteal vein
c. Semimembranous forms the medial border
d. To palpate the popliteal pulse the knee should be held in extension
e. Common peroneal nerve lies laterally in the popliteal fossa

9.7 **Regarding the sciatic nerve:**

a. It supplies the calf muscles via the tibial nerve
b. Injury causes loss of the ankle jerk reflex
c. Derived from L4–S3
d. Supplies sensation to the lateral side of the foot
e. Supplies the hamstring and superficial peroneal muscles

9.8 **Regarding the ulnar nerve:**

a. At the wrist it lies between the scaphoid and hook of the hamate
b. Supplies the abductor pollicis brevis
c. Tinel's sign is positive in ulnar nerve palsy
d. Supplies the brachioradialis
e. Supplies the two medial lumbricals in the hand

9.9 **Regarding the ulnar nerve:**

a. Palsy causes wasting in the first dorsal web space
b. Derived from the anterior cord of the brachial plexus
c. Injury to the medial epicondyle is associated with ulnar nerve damage
d. Froment's test is positive in palsy
e. Supplies the two lateral lumbricals

9.10 **Regarding the radial nerve:**

a. Facilitates wrist extension
b. Is the motor supply to the biceps
c. Monteggia fracture dislocation can cause palsy
d. Long-standing damage can cause 'Simian' thumb
e. Derived from the posterior cord of the brachial plexus

9.11 **Regarding the femoral nerve:**

a. Derived from L2–L4
b. Lies lateral to the femoral artery in the femoral canal
c. Supplies sensation to the lateral and posterior aspects of the thigh
d. Supplies the knee joint
e. Supplies the ankle reflex

9.12 **Regarding vertebral anatomy:**

a. There are eight cervical vertebrae
b. Herniation of the nucleus polposus occurs predominately posteriorly
c. Rotation occurs predominately in the thoracic column
d. There are 12 thoracic vertebrae
e. Conus medullaris lies at the L3 in adulthood

9.13 **Regarding the vertebral level C6:**

a. Bifurcation of the common carotid artery occurs here
b. This is the level of the cricoid cartilage
c. This is the level of the superior border of the scapula
d. This is the level the pharynx becomes the oesophagus
e. This is the level the inferior thyroid artery crosses the thyroid gland

9.14 **Regarding skull foramina:**

a. Cranial nerve X exits via the jugular foramen
b. Cranial nerve V exits via the foramen ovale
c. Middle meningeal vessels exit via the foramen spinosum
d. Accessory nerve exits via the jugular foramen
e. External jugular vein transverses the jugular foramen

9.15 **Regarding vertebral levels:**

a. Oesophageal opening in the diaphragm is at T10
b. Aortic opening in the diaphragm is at T8
c. Upper border of the liver is at T4
d. L1 is the level of the fundus of the gallbladder
e. L1 is the level of the hilum of the spleen

9.16 **Regarding the optic nerve:**

a. Injury to the left optic tract causes a left homonymous hemianopia
b. Injury to the optic chiasma causes a bitemporal hemianopia
c. Injury to the right optic nerve causes a right homonymous hemianopia
d. Pituitary adenoma is associated with optic chiasma injury
e. The optic nerve terminates in the lateral geniculate body

9.17 **Regarding Ludwig's angina:**

a. Treatment involves the use of glycerol trinitrate spray
b. Infection commences in the pre-auricular area
c. Causes include IV drug abuse
d. Causes include retropharyngeal abscess
e. Causes coronary artery spasm

9.18   Regarding tissue spaces in the neck:

a. Parapharyngeal space is a continuation of the retropharyngeal space
b. Submandibular space contains the mylohyoid muscle
c. Retropharyngeal space lies immediately anterior to the prevertebral fascia
d. Retropharyngeal space extends to the diaphragm
e. Prevertebral space communicates with the axilla

9.19   Regarding the anatomy of the trachea:

a. It bifurcates at the level of the suprasternal notch
b. Lined by squamous epithelium
c. Thymus gland lies anterior
d. Recurrent laryngeal nerves lie anteriorly
e. Is supplied by the inferior thyroid artery

9.20   Regarding the cranial nerves:

a. Hypoglossal nerve supplies the tongue
b. Maxillary nerve supplies the tongue
c. Accessory nerve has cranial and spinal roots
d. Accessory nerve supplies the deltoid muscle
e. Accessory nerve exits the skull via the jugular foramen

9.21   Regarding cranial nerve palsies:

a. Paralysis of the superior rectus muscle causes diplopia on looking upwards
b. A fourth nerve palsy causes failure of lateral eye movement
c. A third nerve palsy causes a convergent strabismus
d. A sixth cranial nerve palsy causes failure of medial eye movement and a convergent strabismus
e. A third cranial nerve palsy causes complete ptosis

9.22   Regarding lumbar puncture:

a. If the patient is seated there is a greater chance of herniation
b. Posterior spinous process lies at the same level as the L4 spinous process
c. Needle is felt to 'give' when the skin is pierced
d. CSF should be aspirated
e. Post-lumbar puncture headache usually settles with bed rest and analgesia

9.23   Regarding the inguinal region:

a. Superficial inguinal ring is an opening in the external oblique aponeurosis
b. Spermatic cord does not contain the vas deferens
c. Spermatic cord covering is composed partly of the external oblique
d. Spermatic cord has four coverings
e. Testicular artery is part of the spermatic cord

9.24 The following are retroperitoneal structures:

a. Kidney
b. Third part of the duodenum
c. Inferior vena cava
d. Ureter
e. Spleen

9.25 The posterior relations of the duodenum:

a. Bile duct is posterior to the first part of the duodenum
b. Pancreas is posterior to the first part of the duodenum
c. Hepatic artery is posterior to the second part of the duodenum
d. Hilum of the right kidney is posterior to the second part of the duodenum
e. Aorta is posterior to the second part of the duodenum

9.26 Regarding the arterial supply of the gastrointestinal tract:

a. Inferior mesenteric artery supplies the left two-thirds of the transverse colon
b. Inferior mesenteric artery lies posterior to the third part of the duodenum
c. Common hepatic artery is a branch of the coeliac artery
d. Splenic artery is a branch of the superior mesenteric artery
e. Coeliac trunk arises at T12

9.27 Femoral triangle boundaries:

a. Psoas, pectineus, and adductor longus form the floor
b. Inguinal ligament lies laterally
c. Lateral border of adductor longus lies medially
d. Medial border of sartorius lies laterally
e. Contains the deep inguinal lymph nodes

9.28 Inguinal triangle boundaries:

a. Inguinal ligament lies inferiorly
b. Inferior epigastric artery lies medially
c. It contains Cloquet's node
d. Lacunar ligament lies medially
e. Lateral edge of rectus abdominus lies medially

9.29 Foramen of Winslow:

a. Contains the superior mesenteric artery
b. Second part of the duodenum lies inferiorly
c. Caudate lobe of the liver lies superiorly
d. Portal vein lies anteriorly
e. Inferior vena cava lies anteriorly

9.30   **Regarding the internal carotid artery:**

a. Is the source of the ophthalmic artery
b. Is the source of the anterior communicating artery
c. Enters the skull through the stylomastoid foramen
d. Is the source of the posterior cerebral artery
e. Supplies the frontal cortex

9.31   **Regarding the common carotid artery:**

a. It is crossed by the facial nerve
b. Supplies the facial artery and lingual artery
c. Internal carotid artery lies medial to the middle ear in the petrous temporal bone
d. Internal carotid artery divides into the middle and posterior cerebral arteries
e. Inferior thyroid artery is the lowest branch of the external carotid artery

9.32   **Regarding internal jugular vein anatomy:**

a. Runs posterolaterally to the carotid artery
b. Enters the axillary vein
c. Enters the subclavian vein
d. Lies medial to the sternocleidomastoid in the upper part of the neck
e. Enters the vein near to the medial border of the anterior scalene muscle

9.33   **Regarding the subclavian vein anatomy:**

a. Becomes the brachiocephalic
b. Lies anterior to the brachial plexus
c. Internal mammary artery lies medial and anterior to it
d. It joins the external jugular vein
e. Arises from the external jugular vein

9.34   **Regarding the anatomy of the aorta:**

a. It lies anterior to the body of the pancreas
b. Inferior vena cava lies on its left side
c. Superior mesenteric branch arises at L3
d. Divides into the common iliac arteries at L5
e. Lies anterior to the lesser sac

9.35   **Regarding the anatomy of the inferior vena cava:**

a. Is crossed by the portal vein
b. Right renal veins drain directly into it
c. Veins of L3 and L4 drain directly into it
d. Lies to the right of the aorta
e. Penetrates the diaphragm at T6

9.1 Answers

a. **True**
b. **True**
c. **True**
d. **True**
e. **True**

9.2 Answers

a. **True**
b. **False** – the ulnar nerve lies anterior to the carpal tunnel
c. **False** – the ulnar artery lies anterior to the carpal tunnel
d. **False** – the flexor radialis lies anterior and lateral to the carpal tunnel
e. **True**

9.3 Answers

a. **True**
b. **True**
c. **True**
d. **True**
e. **False** – the trunks of the brachial plexus lie at the base of the posterior triangle

9.4 Answers

a. **True**
b. **False** – the sartorius laterally rotates the thigh at the hip joint
c. **True**
d. **False** – the rectus femoris flexes the thigh at the hip joint
e. **False** – the rectus femoris is innervated by the femoral nerve

9.5 Answers

a. **True**
b. **True**
c. **False** – the gluteus maximus is innervated by the inferior gluteal nerve
d. **True**
e. **True**

9.6 Answers

a. **True**
b. **False** – the tibial nerve lies superficial to the popliteal vein
c. **True**
d. **False** – the knee should be flexed to allow deep palpation
e. **True**

9.7 Answers

a. **True**
b. **True**
c. **True**
d. **True**
e. **True**

9.8 Answers

a. **False** – at the wrist the ulnar nerve lies between the pisiform and the hook of the hamate
b. **False** – the abductor pollicis brevis is supplied by the median nerve
c. **False** – Tinel's sign is a test for median nerve palsy in patients with carpal tunnel syndrome
d. **False** – the brachioradialis is supplied by the radial nerve
e. **True**

9.9 Answers

a. **True**
b. **False** – the ulnar nerve is derived from the medial cord
c. **True**
d. **True** – Froment's test is a test of the motor function of adductor pollicis used in assessing ulnar nerve function
e. **False** – the ulnar nerve supplies the two medial lumbricals

9.10 Answers

a. **True**
b. **False** – the radial nerve supplies the triceps
c. **True**
d. **False** – 'Simian' thumb occurs post damage to the median nerve
e. **True**

9.11 Answers

a. **True**
b. **True**
c. **False** – the femoral nerve supplies sensation to the medial and anterior thigh
d. **True**
e. **False** – the sciatic nerve supplies the ankle reflex

9.12 Answers

a. **False** - there are seven cervical vertebrae
b. **True**
c. **True**
d. **True**
e. **False** – the conus medullaris lies at level of L1 or L2 in adulthood and at L3 at birth

9.13 Answers

a. **False** – bifurcation of the common carotid artery occurs at C4
b. **True**
c. **False** – T2 is the level of the superior border of the scapula
d. **True**
e. **True**

9.14 Answers

a. **True** – the vagus nerve
b. **True** – the mandibular branch
c. **True**
d. **True**
e. **False** – the internal jugular vein traverses the jugular foramen

9.15 Answers

a. **True**
b. **False** – the aortic opening in the diaphragm is at T12
c. **False** – the upper border of the liver is at T6
d. **True**
e. **True**

9.16 Answers

a. **False** – injury to the left optic tract causes a right homonymous hemianopia
b. **True**
c. **False** – injury to the right optic nerve causes a blind right eye
d. **True** – due to local compression
e. **True**

9.17 Answers

a. **False** – Ludwig's angina is due to a bacterial infection
b. **False** – infection generally commences in the sublingual or submaxillary spaces
c. **True**
d. **True**
e. **False**

9.18 Answers

a. **True** – the parapharyngeal space is a lateral extension of the retropharyngeal space
b. **True**
c. **True**
d. **True** – the retropharyngeal space extends to the diaphragm via the anterior and posterior mediastinum
e. **True**

9.19 Answers

a. **False** – the trachea bifurcates at the level of the manubriosternal notch
b. **False** – the trachea is lined by pseudostratified columnar epithelium
c. **True**
d. **False** – the recurrent laryngeal nerves lie posterior to the trachea
e. **True**

9.20 Answers

a. **True**
b. **True**
c. **True**
d. **False** – the accessory nerve supplies the sternocleidomastoid and the trapezius
e. **True** – the accessory nerve exits the skull via the jugular foramen with the glossopharyngeal and vagus nerves

9.21 Answers

a. **True**
b. **False** – a lesion of the fourth nerve causes weak downwards and outwards eye movement
c. **False** – a third nerve palsy causes a divergent strabismus
d. **False** – a sixth cranial nerve palsy causes failure of lateral eye movement and a divergent strabismus
e. **True**

9.22 Answers

a. **True**
b. **True**
c. **False** – the needle is felt to 'give' when the dura is pierced
d. **False** – CSF should be allowed to drain; if aspirated a nerve root may be trapped against the needle and injured
e. **True**

9.23 Answers

a. **True**
b. **False**
c. **True** – the external spermatic fascia is derived from the external oblique
d. **False** – the spermatic cord has three coverings: the external spermatic fascia, the cremasteric fascia, and internal spermatic fascia
e. **True**

9.24 Answers

a. **True**
b. **False** – the second part of the duodenum is retroperitoneal
c. **True**
d. **True**
e. **False**

9.25 Answers

a. **True**
b. **True**
c. **False** – the hepatic artery is posterior to the first part of the duodenum
d. **True**
e. **False** – the aorta is posterior to the third part of the duodenum

9.26 Answers

a. **False** – the inferior mesenteric artery supplies the left one-third of the transverse colon
b. **True**
c. **True**
d. **False** – the splenic artery is a branch of the coeliac artery
e. **True**

9.27 Answers

a. **True**
b. **False** – the inguinal ligament forms the superior boundary
c. **False** – the medial border of the adductor longus lies medially
d. **True**
e. **True**

9.28 Answers

a. **True**
b. **False** – the inferior epigastric artery lies laterally
c. **False** – Cloquet's node is in the femoral ring
d. **False** – the lacunar ligament lies on the floor of the inguinal triangle; it supports the medial border
e. **True**

9.29 Answers

a. **False**
b. **False** – the first part of the duodenum lies inferiorly to the foramen of Winslow
c. **True**
d. **True**
e. **False** – the inferior vena cava lies posterior to the foramen of Winslow

9.30 Answers

a. **True**
b. **False** – the internal carotid artery is the source of the posterior communicating artery
c. **False** – the internal carotid artery enters through the carotid canal
d. **False** – the posterior cerebral artery is formed by the bifurcation of the basilar artery
e. **True**

9.31 Answers

a. **True** – the common carotid artery is crossed by the facial nerve in the parotid gland
b. **True**
c. **True**
d. **False** – the internal carotid artery divides into the anterior and middle cerebral arteries
e. **False** – the lowest branch of the external carotid artery is the superior thyroid artery

9.32 Answers

a. **True**
b. **False**
c. **True**
d. **True**
e. **True**

9.33 Answers

a. **True**
b. **True**
c. **False** – the internal mammary artery lies posterior to the subclavian vein
d. **False** – the subclavian vein unites with the internal jugular vein
e. **False** – the axillary vein becomes the subclavian vein which unites with the internal jugular vein to become the brachiocephalic vein

9.34 Answers

a. ~~**True**~~ *False*
b. **False** – the inferior vena cava lies on its right side
c. **False** – the superior mesenteric branch arises at L1
d. **False** – the aorta divides into the common iliac arteries at L4
e. **True** *False*

9.35 Answers

a. **True**
b. **True**
c. **True**
d. **True**
e. **False** – the inferior vena cava passes through the caval opening at T8